Assessing Evidence to Improve Population Health and Wellbeing

Titles in the Series

Policy and Strategy for Improving Health and Wellbeing ISBN 9780857250070
Leadership and Collaborative Working in Public Health ISBN 9780857252906
Measuring Health and Wellbeing ISBN 9780857254337

To order, please contact our distributor: BEBC Distribution, Albion Close, Parkstone, Poole, BH12 3LL. Telephone: 0845 230 9000, email: learningmatters@bebc.co.uk. You can also find more information on each of these titles and our other learning resources at www.learningmatters.co.uk

Assessing Evidence to Improve Population Health and Wellbeing

Editor: Carmen Aceijas

Series Editor:
Vicki Taylor

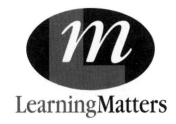

LearningMatters

First published in 2011 by Learning Matters Ltd

British Library Cataloguing in Publication Data
A CIP record for this book is available from the British Library.
ISBN 9780857253897

This book is also available in the following ebook formats:
Adobe ebook ISBN: 9780857253910
EPUB ebook ISBN: 9780857253903
Kindle ISBN: 9780857253927

Cover and text design by Code 5 Design Associates
Project management by Swales & Willis Ltd, Exeter, Devon
Typeset by Swales & Willis Ltd, Exeter, Devon
Printed and bound in Great Britain by Short Run Press Ltd, Exeter, Devon

Learning Matters Ltd
20 Cathedral Yard
Exeter EX1 1HB
Tel: 01392 215560
info@learningmatters.co.uk
www.learningmatters.co.uk

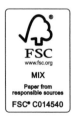

FSC
www.fsc.org
MIX
Paper from
responsible sources
FSC® C014540

Contents

Foreword from the Series Editor

The publication of the Public Health Skills and Career Framework in April 2008 provided, for the first time, an overall framework for career development in public health in the United Kingdom. Prior to this, the focus had been primarily on the public health specialist workforce. The development of the Framework itself was a truly collaborative enterprise involving a large number of organisations and stakeholder groups and was designed to enable individuals at any stage of their career to identify a pathway for skills and career progression.

Within the Framework, public health is divided into nine areas of work. There are four core areas that anyone working in public health must know about and have certain competences within. There are five non-core or 'defined' areas, representing the contexts within which individuals principally work and develop.

Core areas	Non-core (defined) areas
Surveillance and assessment of the population's health and wellbeing	Health improvement
	Health protection
Assessing the evidence of effectiveness of interventions, programmes and services	Public health intelligence
Policy and strategy development and implementation	Academic public health
Leadership and collaborative working	Health & Social Care Quality

This new series, 'Transforming Public Health Practice', has been developed as a direct response to the development of the Framework and has a book dedicated to each of the four core areas of public health: Measuring health and wellbeing; Assessing evidence to improve population health and wellbeing; Policy and strategy for improving health and wellbeing; and Leadership and collaborative working for health and wellbeing are all featured.

The Framework defines nine levels of competence and knowledge: Level 1 will have little previous knowledge, skills or experience in public health, while those at level 9 will be setting strategic priorities and direction and providing leadership to improve population health and wellbeing. This series is aimed at those who want to develop their skills and knowledge in public health at levels 7–9 (which broadly equates to Masters level) although the series will be relevant to a wider group with the publication of the Public Health Practitioner standards (UKPHR) and opening of the Public Health Practitioner Register (UKPHR). This will include those interested in acquiring or developing their public health competences and knowledge and, in particular, those who are seeking to demonstrate their public health skills and knowledge (and may be considering putting together a portfolio to demonstrate this, at specialist or practitioner level).

This series will also be useful for anyone whose work involves improving people's health and wellbeing, or has a direct impact on the health and wellbeing of communities and populations – this encompasses a wide range of work areas and of organisations and agencies.

Individual books in the series outline the key knowledge and skills in the core area and take these further through case studies and scenarios how these competences can be used in practice. It is hoped that activities and self-assessment tools provided throughout the books will help the reader to hone their critical thinking and reflection skills.

Chapters in each of the books follow a standard format. At the beginning a box highlights links to relevant competences. This sets the scene and enables the reader to see exactly what will be covered. This is extended by a chapter overview, which sets out the key topics and what the reader should expect to have learnt by the end of the chapter.

There is usually at least one case study in each chapter, which considers public health skills and knowledge in practice. Activities such as practical tasks with learning points, critical thinking and reflective practice are also included. Each activity is followed by a brief commentary on issues raised. At the end of each chapter a summary provides a reminder of what has been covered.

All chapters are evidence based in that they set out theory or evidence that underpins practice. A list of additional readings is set out under the 'Going further' section, with all references collated at the end of the book.

In summary, this series will provide invaluable support to anyone studying or practising in the field of public health, in a range of different settings.

Vicki Taylor
Independent Public Health Consultant & Director,
The Roundhouse Consultancy, MK Ltd.
Associate Lecturer, The Open University
Previously Senior Lecturer, London Southbank University,
Senior Lecturer, Kings College, London

Author Information

Dr Carmen Aceijas graduated in psychology and finished her PhD in research and methods [health psychology] in 2005. She has worked in research and academia in public health since 1998 for institutions such the University of East London, London School of Hygiene & Tropical Medicine, Imperial College and Andalusian School of Public Health. During the last 12 years she has been working in public health research on drug dependences and HIV. Currently Carmen is a senior lecturer in public health in the University of East London (Stratford) and programme leader of the postgraduate programmes in public health and health promotion.

Amina Dilmohamed is currently working as a senior lecturer in public health at the University of East London (Stratford). She has a background in clinical education and research, and is currently lecturing in undergraduate and postgraduate public health modules and supervises students for their dissertation at both levels.

Dr Nena Foster is a senior lecturer in public health and the BSc (Hons) public health programme leader at the University of East London (Stratford). She has lectured and researched in the UK and abroad in areas of health, social policy, social exclusion and multiculturalism. Her current research involves exploring the health and social implications of ageing with HIV. She has also supervised a number of students in projects related to HIV and other areas of health.

Gary Ginsberg attained a DrPH from UNC. He was employed by the Institute of Psychiatry and Wandsworth Borough before moving to be director of medical technology assessment sector of the Israeli Ministry of Health. He specialises in evaluating potential interventions using cost–utility analysis. He recently spent two years with the WHO in Geneva and has published over 90 articles. More importantly, the adoption of some of the articles' conclusions has led to the saving of many lives.

Dr Mahwish Hayee has a background in medicine and started her teaching career in the field of public health. She is currently a lecturer in public health at University of East London (Stratford), where she is responsible for teaching undergraduate and postgraduate students. She has a special interest in infectious diseases and global issues in public health.

Dr Krishna R. Regmi is a lecturer in public health at University of East London (Stratford). He is engaged in teaching and research in public health, with special interest in health services/systems research. His previous research and publications include health sector reform, health inequalities, inter-professional education, and gender and health both internationally and in the UK.

Introduction
Carmen Aceijas

Public health interventions and programmes are accountable, as are any other aspect of the practices around health issues, for their capacity to produce sound evidence on their virtues and limitations. This book explores the different approaches to understanding, assessing and improving the evidence emerging from the careful examination of public health actions.

In this sense, it is a suitable tool for practitioners and specialists in public health who wish to improve their knowledge of how public health is granted with the required qualification of evidence-based public health and how it links to the improvement of the health and wellbeing of the population.

The timing of this book is especially relevant as it appears shortly after the publication of the UK government White Paper for Public Health, which contains numerous acknowledgements of the tremendous contribution of public health to the health of UK: 'Most of the major advances in life expectancy over the last two centuries came from public health rather than health care' (Department of Health, 2010, page 11). The government's ambitious and revolutionary strategy places public health at the centre of the health agenda; 'It is time to prioritise public health' (page 26) and consequently, with the major organisational and functional re-shift of the public health functions proposed in the document, attention is provided to its workforce. Thus, the White Paper clearly spells out that supportive funding will be provided to fulfil the commitments made in the document: 'The Government will ring-fence public health funds from within the overall NHS budget to ensure that it is prioritised' (Department of Health, 2010, pages 26, 51, 57; Department of Health–NHS, 2010, page 5).

The need for a strong, well-trained public health workforce is recognised in the White Paper as part of its strategic plan: 'We envisage that the public health workforce will be known for its expertise – public health staff, whatever their discipline and wherever they work, will be well-trained and expert in their field' (Department of Health, 2010, page 71). It provides several examples where specific inputs will be needed (e.g. further 4200 health visitors, development of specialist workforce for public health information and intelligence and so on) and presents a vision of empowered and well-motivated public health practitioners from all sectors, including health care (Department of Health, 2010, page 60).

These are, therefore, good times to invest in training and this book is an excellent tool that, as part of the series 'Transforming Public Health Practice', aims to help students to approach the specific expertise surrounding evidence in public health. Throughout the book, readers will learn the main theoretical concepts that can equip them with good strong foundations in the area, and the theoretical knowledge will be developed further to provide an understanding of how the assessment of evidence is pursued, constructed and disseminated in a variety of scenarios.

For practitioners, this will enable them to examine and act with a critical and systematic eye when contributing to design and implementation of public health interventions. At the specialist level, this book will prove to be a valuable tool for those in charge of managerial duties in public health, from the commissioning of services to the formal evaluation of interventions.

Is this book for me?

This book addresses the core standards for public health practice as defined by the UK Department of Health in the UK Public Health Skills and Career Framework (UK PHSCF) (Department of Health, 2008). It covers the second core area of the Framework – 'Assessing the evidence of effectiveness of interventions, programmes and services to improve population health and wellbeing' – as an area of practice that 'focuses on the critical assessment of evidence relating to the effectiveness and cost-effectiveness of health and wellbeing and related interventions, programmes and services, and the application to practice through planning, audit and evaluation' (Department of Health, 2008, page 18).

In this sense, the primary aim of the authors was to create a practical tool for those learning or interested in how evidence is assessed in public health and to acquire specialist knowledge on its methodologies, applications, extent and limitations. Case studies and activities are drawn from international knowledge and examples of public health interventions around the world, and have been designed to provide real scenarios where both conceptual and procedural aspects of evidence in public health can be applied. Thus the reader can easily move from theory to practice by studying the numerous examples of how to generate and assess evidence in public health included here.

How the book works

The book is divided into nine chapters with each chapter exploring different aspects of evidence in public health from the definition and analysis of its main concepts to the application to specific scenarios.

All chapters cover different knowledge contents at levels 4–8 of the UK PHSCF (Department of Health, 2008, pages 19–21) but especially knowledge contents in level 7. Such knowledge content aims to build a set of competences in this area. At level 7 such competences are:

1. *Critically appraise and summarise evidence from a range of sources*
2. *Formulate recommendations for change on the basis of critically appraised evidence*
3. *Influence the development of policies, procedures, guidelines or protocols on the basis of critically appraised evidence*
4. *Advise a range of audiences about evidence*

5. *Identify gaps in evidence and initiate action to fill these gaps*
6. *Review own area of work to ensure it is effective in achieving its aims.*

(Public Health Skills and Careers Framework, Department
of Health, 2008, page 20)

Therefore, this book is a critical tool in acquiring the set of competences as outlined
by the Department of Health.

The first chapter covers the main concepts and the theoretical development of evidence-based public health; the following four chapters enable students to understand
evidence mainly from written sources and help them to develop skills to critically
appraise different forms of scientific information, enabling them to assess whether
and up to what point the knowledge around a given topic can be qualified as evidence.
The final four chapters cover more specific and specialised areas of public health, intimately linked to efforts to assess the benefits of programmes and interventions.

How to use this book

An examination of the UK PHSCF will provide you with a good understanding of the
competences you have to acquire or improve upon in your progress as a public health
practitioner or specialist and how they match with the National Occupational Standards for public health. If you know the topic you want to study (or competence you
wish to focus on), look at the table below, which gives you a quick guide to the chapter
titles and competences. These relate to competences set out in the Public Health Skills
and Careers Framework, the Public Health Practitioner Standards and National Occupational Standards for public health, as covered within the chapter. This is an easy
way to locate the chapters you should be reading according to the competence you are
aiming to master at each point of your learning process. A chapter overview, at the
beginning of each chapter, augments this information and sets you in the right direction. If used in the context of a formally directed course in public health, the map-
ping of competences aims to provide a meaningful understanding on why contents
are introduced in such a training and what their ultimate goal is. At the end of the
day, they all are directed to the ultimate goal of training the public health workforce
according to transparent and nationally acknowledged standards. Be a part of it!

Table 0.1 Chapters, occupational standards and UK PHSCF levels (Department of Health, 2008)

Occupational standard	*UK PHSCF – Knowledge*
Chapter 1. What is meant by evidence?	LEVEL 4
HSC33 Reflect on and develop your practice	c) Knowledge of the purpose and
M&L C2 Encourage innovation in your area of	methods of reviewing own area of
responsibility	work and the role of various people in
CJ F309 Support and challenge workers on specific	this
aspects of their practice	LEVEL 5
HI124 Facilitate the clinical audit process	a) Knowledge of literature searching
HI127 Develop evidence based clinical guidelines	techniques

d) Understanding of the purpose and methods of reviewing effectiveness in own area of work

LEVEL 6

a) Understanding of how to search literature

b) Knowledge of the principles of critical appraisal as applied to various studies, and its use in improving health and wellbeing

Chapter 2. What are sources of evidence?

HSC33 Reflect on and develop your practice

M&L C2 Encourage innovation in your area of responsibility

CJ F309 Support and challenge workers on specific aspects of their practice

HI124 Facilitate the clinical audit process

HI125 Search for clinical information and evidence according to an accepted methodology

HI127 Develop evidence based clinical guidelines

LEVEL 6

a) Understanding of how to search literature

b) Knowledge of the principles of critical appraisal as applied to various studies, and its use in improving health and wellbeing

c) Understanding of the levels of evidence and their importance for decision-making in own areas of work

LEVEL 7

b) Understanding of the hierarchy of evidence as it applies to services, programmes and interventions which impact on health and wellbeing

Chapter 3. Making sense of the evidential hierarchy used to judge research evidence

PHS07 Assess the evidence and impact of health and health care interventions, programmes and services and apply the assessments to practice

PHS08 Improve the quality of health and health care interventions and services through audit and evaluation

CJ F309 Support and challenge workers on specific aspects of their practice

LEVEL 6

c) Understand the levels of evidence and their importance for decision-making in own areas of work

LEVEL 7

1 b) Understanding the hierarchy of evidence as it applies to services, programmes and interventions which impact on health and wellbeing

Chapter 4. The act/art of assessing: Critical appraisal and its relevance in public health

PHS07 Assess the evidence and impact of health and health care interventions, programmes and services and apply the assessments to practice

PHS08 Improve the quality of health and health care interventions and services through audit and evaluation

LEVEL 6

b) Knowledge of the principles of critical appraisal as applied to various studies, and its use in improving health and wellbeing

CJ F309 Support and challenge workers on specific aspects of their practice

LEVEL 7
a) Understanding of appraising the quality of primary and secondary research

Chapter 5. Assessing evidence – the quality of primary and secondary research

HSC33 Reflect on and develop your practice
M&L C2 Encourage innovation in your area of responsibility
CJ F309 Support and challenge workers on specific aspects of their practice
HI127 Develop evidence based clinical guidelines
PHP46 Create and capitalise upon opportunities to advocate the need for improving health and wellbeing
PHS11 Communicate effectively with the public and others about improving the health and wellbeing of the population

LEVEL 6
c) Understand the levels of evidence and their importance for decision-making in own areas of work
LEVEL 7
a) Understanding of appraising the quality of primary and secondary research
b) Understanding the hierarchy of evidence as it applies to services, programmes and interventions which impact on health and wellbeing

6. Assessing evidence – the strengths and weaknesses of various ways of assessing public health outcomes

PHS07 Assess the evidence and impact of health and health care interventions, programmes and services and apply the assessments to practice
PHS08 Improve the quality of health and health care interventions and services through audit and evaluation
HP10 Monitor and review effectiveness of services and initiatives to protect health, wellbeing and safety
CJ F309 Support and challenge workers on specific aspects of their practice

LEVEL 6
b) Knowledge of the principles of critical appraisal as applied to various studies, and its use in improving health and wellbeing
LEVEL 7
c) Understanding of the strengths and weaknesses of various ways of assessing outcomes

Chapter 7. Assessing evidence – cost-effectiveness analysis

M&L C2 Encourage innovation in your area of responsibility
HI124 Facilitate the clinical audit process
HI127 Develop evidence based clinical guidelines

LEVEL 6
d) Knowledge of various techniques to assess productivity and cost-effectiveness
LEVEL 7
e) Understanding of the validity and use of various techniques to assess productivity and cost-effectiveness, and the inferences that can be drawn

Chapter 8. Principles and methods of programme evaluation

PHS07 Assess the evidence and impact of health and health care interventions, programmes and services and apply the assessments to practice

PHS08 Improve the quality of health and health care interventions and services through audit and evaluation

CJ F309 Support and challenge workers on specific aspects of their practice

LEVEL 7

d) Knowledge of the principles and methods of evaluation (. . .), as applied to improving quality

Chapter 9. Assessing quality and effectiveness to improve public health and wellbeing

PHS07 Assess the evidence and impact of health and health care interventions, programmes and services and apply the assessments to practice

PHS08 Improve the quality of health and health care interventions and services through audit and evaluation

LEVEL 8

a) Understanding of the principles and methods of evaluation, audit, research and development, and standard setting, as applied to improving quality

chapter 1

What is Meant by Evidence?

Carmen Aceijas and Amina Dilmohamed

Meeting the public health competences

Core area: Assessing the evidence of effectiveness of interventions, programmes and services to improve population health and wellbeing.

This chapter will help you to evidence the following competences for public health (Public Health Skills and Careers Framework):

- Level 5 (a): Knowledge of literature searching techniques
- Level 5 (d): Understanding of the purpose and methods of reviewing effectiveness in own area of work
- Level 6 (a): Understanding of how to search literature
- Level 6 (b): Knowledge of the principles of critical appraisal as applied to various studies, and its use in improving health and wellbeing
- Level 7 (a) Understanding of appraising the quality of primary and secondary research.

This chapter will also assist you in demonstrating the following National Occupational Standard(s) for public health:

- Reflect on and develop your practice – (HSC33)
- Encourage innovation in your area of responsibility – (M&L C2)
- Facilitate the clinical audit process – (HI124)
- Develop evidence based clinical guidelines – (HI127).

This chapter will also be useful in demonstrating Standard 4c and 4e and 7 of the Public Health Practitioner Standards.

- Standard 4. Continually develop and improve own and others' practice in public health by:

    d. the application of evidence in improving own area of work
    e. objectively and constructively contributing to reviewing the effectiveness of own area of work.

- Standard 7. Assess the evidence of effective interventions and services to improve health and wellbeing – demonstrating:

    a. knowledge of the different types, sources and levels of evidence in own area of practice and how to access and use them
    b. the appraisal of published evidence and the identification of implications for own area of work practice.

Chapter overview

This chapter will help you to consider what evidence in public health is, and how it is related to evidence-based public health, its principles, why and when it is needed and its role in the decision making for programmes, interventions and services. Some discussion of its historical development is included to help you to understand how evidence became central to public health and to appreciate why all public health actions should be evidence based. This chapter will help you to develop your thinking about evidence in public health, and in particular the overall approach to the assessment of evidence for different interventions, programmes and services. Exercises in this chapter will focus on:

- developing clarity about the nature and origins of evidence in public health;
- developing a critical awareness of the importance of evidence-based public health for the public in general and, in particular, for stakeholders;
- understanding the key principles of evidence gathering and critical appraisal.

Public health professionals are regularly required to participate in the design and implementation of evidence-based projects and their evaluation. In order to help you to identify ways to identify evidence more effectively, in this chapter the key steps of the process will be explored. A number of useful tools that can be used at each stage are introduced here and further explored in following chapters.

After reading this chapter you will be able to:

- identify the nature and main features of evidence-based public health;
- appreciate and be aware of the origins of the concept;
- demonstrate familiarity with the basic process of gathering information and assessing evidence.

What is evidence-based public health?

Evidence, at the most basic level, involves 'the available body of facts or information indicating whether a belief or proposition is true or valid' (Jewell and Abate, 2001) and from this definition we can start to understand that evidence-based public health is something that allows and aims for the production of a body of facts generated with robust systematically assessed or appraised system(s).

Evidence-based public health is an approach in public health that evolved from evidence-based medicine (EBM), which originated from an early plea to adopt an evidence-based approach in medicine. This plea was the work of the British epidemiologist Archie Cochrane (1909–1988), who in his seminal work *Effectiveness and Efficiency: Random Reflections on Health Services* (Cochrane, 1972), challenged the dominant medical authorities of his time to prove that what they did made any real difference. He further went on to criticise the lack of scientific methods in clinical practice: 'It is surely a great criticism of our profession that we have not organised a critical summary, by speciality or subspecialty, updated periodically, of all relevant randomised controlled trials' (Cochrane, 1979, pages 10–11).

Cochrane's intuitive thoughts instigated the formation of the Cochrane Collaboration in 1992, an international network that synthesises what does and what does not work in health care or, in other words, supplements professional decisions with the latest research knowledge. As Cochrane pointed out many years ago, failing to conduct systematic, up-to-date reviews of controlled trials of health care may result in substantial adverse consequences for patients, practitioners, the health services, researchers and research funding bodies.

Perhaps the most cited author to define evidence-based medicine, however, is David Sackett. He defined evidence-based medicine as:

> *the conscientious, explicit and judicious use of current best evidence in making decisions about the care of individual patients. The practice of evidence-base medicine means integrating individual clinical expertise with the best available external clinical evidence from systematic research.*
>
> (Sackett *et al.*, 1996, pages 71–72)

In the field of public health, a number of broad definitions of evidence-based public health have been formulated and the above statement on the origin of evidence-based public health from evidence-based medicine can be exemplified with the definition of evidence-based public health stated by Jenicek in 1997:

> *the conscientious explicit and judicious use of current best evidence in making decisions about the care of communities and populations in the domain of health protection, disease prevention, health maintenance and improvement.*
>
> (Jenicek, 1997, pages 187–197)

The similarities between Sackett's definition of evidence-based medicine and Jenicek's definition of evidence-based public health are obvious: 'the conscientious explicit and judicious use of current best evidence in making decisions about the care of'. From there, Sackett declares the focus of interest as 'individual patients', while Jenicek states that it is 'communities and populations'.

Similarities and differences between the two definitions could have hardly been better placed; both emphasise the dismissal of random or casual approaches. Both evidence-based medicine and evidence-based public health have to be conscientious and explicit. Nothing is left to chance, rather a systematic approach is clearly suggested. The focuses of interest are, however, very different: individual patients in evidence-based medicine versus communities and populations in evidence-based public health.

Jenicek went on to define evidence-based public health as the appropriate use of current best evidence to make decisions about the care of communities and population in the area of disease prevention and health promotion. He was astute to acknowledge that evidence-based public health had its own unique challenges because of its complex interventions and involvement with multiple communities and their societal issues.

Another definition portrays evidence-based public health as:

the development, implementation, and evaluation of effective programs and policies in public health through application of principles of scientific reasoning, including systematic uses of data and information systems, and appropriate use of behavioral science theory and program planning models.

(Brownson *et al.*, 2003, page 4)

While Jenicek's definition focuses on the need of evidence-based public health covering all the working areas of public health (protection, disease prevention, health maintenance and improvement), Brownson's definition emphasises its applicability to all stages (design, implementation and evaluation) of public health interventions. Thus, the two definitions complete and complement each other. They share a common feature – the acknowledgement that evidence-based public health is the result of a conscious process guided by explicit and systematic reckoning aiming to analyse the strength of a given programme, intervention or service in an explicit and objective manner.

Nevertheless, a common error is made when assumptions about absolute degrees of certainty are attributed to programmes, interventions and so on, qualified as evidence based. It is worthwhile, then, clarifying that evidence-based public health looks for the best evidence currently available although this is not necessarily the final truth and that a large quantity of information does not necessarily mean we have sufficient evidence.

In other words, the development of evidence-based public health interventions is based on the best possible scientific information. Thus, both theoretical and systematic planning approaches are followed, distinctively multidisciplinary problem-solving activities are undertaken, the principles of sound evaluation inherent to evidence-based public health are followed, and the dissemination of results is considered as embedded in the standard activities of evidence-based public health.

A further difficulty in our understanding of what constitutes evidence in public health is the variety of forms used to gather evidence depending on the activity we aim to appraise. The traditional understanding and application of evidence in public health referred to the appraisal of findings of research in public health with a medical and biological focus. But the traditional approach to the assessment of evidence by analysing research findings only and within the strict constraints of the scientific method fell short. Since then, the concept has been broadened to cover all public health activities. Both new methodological and theoretical frameworks had to be constructed to enable the analysis of evidence in topics and issues that hardly conformed to the traditional research efforts in biomedical sciences.

Nowadays in public health, evidence is considered to be some form of data including epidemiologic (quantitative) data, results of programme or policy evaluations, and qualitative data for uses in making judgements or decisions. Public health evidence is usually the result of a complex cycle of observation, theory, and experiment (McQueen and Anderson, 2001; Rimer *et al.*, 2001).

Key features of evidence-based public health

The key features of evidence-based public health have been outlined as:

- *conceptual plausibility;*
- *use of different types of evidence to determine what works for whom and in what circumstances;*
- *translation of evidence into practical guidance for policy and practice.*

(Killoran and Kelly, 2010, page xxii)

Conceptual plausibility in evidence-based public health refers to the assumption that we can identify and understand causal relationships between factors influencing health status and the potential interventions. It is closely related to the social model of health that incorporates the role of social determinants in addressing health inequalities with its underlying acknowledgement that the health status can be altered by both modification of external factors and the provision of adequate interventions.

The use of different types of evidence is necessary in searching from the levels of evidence available. Earlier models of evidence-based public health identified scientific research solely as the source of evidence. However, it is acknowledged nowadays than other sources of information, for example clinical observations, must also be taken into account.

Finally, the translation of evidence into practical guidance for policy and practice highlights the clear applicability of the discipline. Thus, gathering evidence is not seen as a knowledge-generating exercise but as activities aiming to inform, shape and modify both policy and practice and taking into consideration specific cultural contexts. The same way, generating evidence-based public health policies and interventions is bound to the findings regarding evidence. Such findings cannot be ignored but are the foundations of credibility, acceptability and effectiveness of any programme, intervention or policy within the field of evidence-based public health.

From the above it seems almost redundant to articulate when it is especially important to use an evidence-based approach. The obvious answer would be 'always'. Nevertheless, it is useful to list some of the activities which should always be underpinned by such an approach:

- when scientific evidence must support decision making;

- to evaluate the effectiveness and cost benefits of public health programmes;

- to implement new public health programmes or interventions;

- when new policies must be established;

- to conduct literature reviews for grant projects.

The use of evidence in public health has enabled its transformation into evidence-based public health, which has brought multiple advantages and strengths to our discipline:

- It enables the decision-making processes to be based on scientific evidence and effective practices. Too often decision-making processes have been based on history, anecdotes and pure pressure from policy makers, which limits the chances of success. Supporting health decisions by evidence and effective practices enhances the likelihood of success.

- It facilitates the retrieval of up-to-date and reliable information about what works and does not work for a given public health issue.

- It reassures on the efficiency of public health measures implemented.

Case study 1.1: A national framework for developing an evidence-based tobacco control programme. The Israeli experience

Healthy Israel 2020 was created in 2005 to develop national health targets and recommend evidence-based interventions to achieve them. The aim was achieved by a multi-stage process aiming at identifying a set of interventions that would be implemented to reach their health targets. The process was designed as follows:

- Evidence-based interventions were to be selected from various sources, including the Cochrane Collaboration, the US Preventive Services Task Force, the US Task Force on Community Preventive Services, and other literature reviews and original studies, ranked by level of evidence.
- Interventions were to be selected from the resultant list based on current patterns of tobacco use in Israel, feasibility of implementation, and the existing political constraints.
- The items were to be prioritised on the basis of their potential future impact, quality of the evidence of effectiveness, and their generalizability as gleaned from the scientific literature. The information from the scientific literature was to be complemented by local evidence and the Committee's expert opinion on feasibility of implementation. Cost, cost-effectiveness, and issues of inequality were also to be considered.

(From Rosen et al., 2010, page 17)

ACTIVITY 1.1

After reading Case study 1.1:

1. Do you think that the multi-stage process followed the key features of evidence-based public health? Why and to what extent?
2. Can you identify the uses of evidence based approach that were utilised in this process?
3. Reflect on how the advantages and strengths of evidence-based public health are exemplified in the Israeli initiative.
4. Spend a few minutes thinking about these questions and write down your answers

How to gather evidence?

The first question when identifying a potential health issue, a gap of knowledge in its understanding or envisioning ways to improve policies, programmes and interventions addressing such health issue is to learn what is already known about it. It might be that the problem has already been identified, the gap of knowledge already filled, the potential improvement of an intervention suggested elsewhere, etc. Therefore, the process of gathering evidence will aim to learn more about it, learn what is already known. It will involve conducting a literature review.

Such process, however natural and basic it may feel, must be carried out in a systematic way. Thus, the process starts with searching for evidence-based public health literature. A model of seven generic steps has been suggested (Brownson *et al.*, 2003, page 128) as follows:

- Step 1: Determine the public health problem and define the question

- Step 2: Select information sources

- Step 3: Identify key concepts and terms

- Step 4: Conduct the search in subject-appropriate databases

- Step 5: Select documents for review

- Step 6: Abstract relevant information from the documentation

- Step 7: Summarise and apply the literature review.

Step 1: Determine the public health problem and define the question

The determination of a public health problem and the definition of the research question will involve the identification of the patient/population experiencing the problem, the intervention or item of interest of the question, the comparison vector to be identified and the expected outcome. This is what is commonly known as the PICO (Patient, Intervention, Comparator, and Outcome) model. When these key parameters have been identified, the research question will easily emerge.

Step 1: Example

There is mounting evidence that the number of overweight and obese children in the UK is growing and that there are programmes specifically designed to help children experiencing overweight problems to adopt regular exercise routines. You are the head of a school with a standard exercise programme but you can see that there are a relevant number of children in your school already experiencing weight problems. You would like to trial one of those specific programmes in your school to reduce the number of children who are overweight and obese but you need the funding for such a programme.

Therefore, you will need to find the supporting evidence for this new programme to obtain the funding.

- Patient population problem: overweight and obese children (P)
- Intervention/item of interest: programme to help children experiencing overweight problems to adopt regular exercise routines (I)
- Comparison: standard exercise programme vs. new programme (C)
- Outcome: reduce the number of children overweight and obese in your school (O)

Research question: Is the new programme to promote regular exercise routines among overweight and obese children effective in reducing the number of overweight and obese children?

Step 2: Select information sources

The different sources of information, their uses and capacities to generate evidence and the different levels of evidence are discussed in Chapter 2. Here suffice to say that selection of appropriate information sources is key to ensuring that your review will produce reliable information on what is known about your question. The selection must be topic and context sensitive. Thus, in the example used here, sources of information from biomedical research facilitating access to formal research studies (empirical research, systematic literature reviews, meta-analysis, etc.), best practice publications and reports produced by previous implementations of similar programmes should be included.

Step 3: Identify key concepts and terms

From the initial identification of parameters in step 1 we will derive a list of key concepts and terms.

Step 3: Example

- **Patient population problem:** overweight and obese children 6–12 years old.
- **Intervention/item of interest:** new programme to help children experiencing overweight problems to adopt regular exercise routines.

Key concepts:

Population problem:	Intervention of interest:
Children	Exercise
Age	Physical activity
School children	Regular exercise
Overweight children	Routine exercise
Obese children	Effective programmes

Programme development
Programme evaluation
Effective programmes

- **Patient population problem:** overweight and obese children 6–12 years old
- **Intervention/item of interest:** new programme to help children experiencing overweight problems to adopt regular exercise routines
- **Comparison:** standard exercise programme vs. new programme
- **Outcome:** reduce the number of children overweight and obese in your school.

Step 4: Conduct the search in subject-appropriate databases

Nowadays there is a sometimes overwhelming number of databases that can be accessed to find information in public health, but the databases to be searched will depend on the topic of our search and we will consider both *sensitivity* (databases that contain a great number of sources of information on our topic of interest) and *specificity* (databases that contain information well within our topic of interest). There are many consolidated databases in public health, for example Cochrane Collaboration and PubMed, as well as others that are more subject specific. The inclusion of databases must follow the principle of saturation: include databases until only duplicates of already identified pieces of information are found.

Step 5: Select documents for review

The selection of documents aims to identify those that are truly relevant to our research question, but when does an 'identified' document become a 'selected' document?

Step 5: Example

Consider the following extract from the abstract of a paper by Salcedo Aguilar et al. (2010, pages 36–42):

> **Objective**: To assess the impact of a two-year recreational physical activity program in 1044 fourth- and fifth-grade primary schoolchildren from the Province of Cuenca, Spain.
>
> **Study design**: Cluster-randomized controlled trial with 10 intervention and 10 control schools. The program consisted of 3 90-minute sessions of physical activity per week, during 28 weeks every year. Changes in endpoints between baseline (September 2004) and the end of follow-up (June 2006) were compared between the control and intervention group[...].
>
> **Results**: Compared with control subjects, intervention girls reduced the frequency of overweight[...]. However, intervention was associated with an increase in the percentage of body fat in boys.[...]
>
> **Conclusion**: In 2 years, the physical activity program lowered the frequency of overweight in girls.

Should this 'identified' document become a 'selected' document? Some of the points to consider in taking this decision will include:

- The paper reports on a programme implemented in Spain. Are cultural differences relevant in this case? Could similar findings have been found if the study had been done in the UK?
- The paper reports on a '2-year recreational physical activity program in fourth- and fifth-grade primary schoolchildren' and 'the program consisted of 3 90-minute sessions of physical activity per week, during 28 weeks every year'. With this information, little is known on the characteristics of the programme. We need further reading of the paper to assess its applicability to our desired programme.
- The paper seems to be methodologically strong. If the characteristics of the programme are comparable to the sort of programme we would like to have in our school, the evidence provided by this paper could be important and, therefore, it should be included in our final review.
- The paper reports on positive findings for girls but not for boys. What could be the reasons?

We need further reading of the paper. However, even if the results were not positive for boys, if the relevance of the study is good, the paper must be selected.

Step 6: Abstract relevant information from the documentation

Step 6 directly relates to the data extraction process, which is generically defined as the process by which researchers obtain the necessary information about study characteristics and findings from the included studies (Centre for Reviews and Dissemination, 2009) and it is a delicate stage where the quality of the review can easily be compromised.

The first principle is that the data extraction system will be defined a priori and applied to all the documents selected. However, in practice, the achievement of this principle will largely depend on the homogeneity of the documents selected. Thus, while it will be safe to expect that quantification of results in terms of change of outcome variables will be included in research papers, best practice documents might not necessarily include such detailed information.

Aside from these considerations, the core of a literature review will be the information extracted from each of the documents and, given the large amount of documents usually included in a review, we will need a standardised data extraction electronic form (Higgins and Deeks, 2008) that provides consistency.

Step 6: Example of data extraction form suitable for our search

Identification features of the study:
- Author
- Article title
- Type of publication (e.g. journal article, conference abstract).

Study characteristics:
- Aim/objectives of the study
- Study design
- Recruitment procedures used (e.g. details of randomisation, blinding).

Participant characteristics at the beginning of the study:
- Age
- Gender
- Ethnicity
- Socio-economic status
- Weight characteristics
- Number of participants in each characteristic category for intervention and control group(s) or mean/median characteristic values.

Intervention and setting:
- Setting in which the intervention is delivered
- Description of the intervention(s) and control(s)
- Description of co-interventions.

Outcome data/results:
- Unit of assessment/analysis
- Statistical techniques used for each pre-specified outcome:
- Measurement tool or method used
- Length of follow-up.

For all intervention group(s) and control group(s):
- Number of participants enrolled
- Number of participants included in analysis
- Number of withdrawals, exclusions, lost to follow-up
- Summary outcome data (dichotomous: number of events, etc. Continuous: mean and standard deviation)
- Results of study analysis (odds ratio, risk ratio and confidence intervals, *P*-value)
  (Adapted from Centre for Reviews and Disseminations, 2009, pages 30–31)

Step 7: Summarise and apply the literature review

In the last step the information generated by the selected documents is appraised and the results evaluated. The appraisal of evidence is dealt with in-depth in the following chapters, but the answer to the question of how strong is the evidence provided by the documents reviewed will determine our capability to answer common questions after conducting a literature review, such as:

- What are the results?

- Are the results valid?

- Were all important outcomes considered?

- Can the results be applied to my context?

Critical appraisal and its role in evidence-based public health

Following the seven steps above will not guarantee in itself that you will acquire the evidence needed but you will have the relevant information. To ascertain the usefulness of the information gathered the process needs to be followed by critical appraisal of the information selected. Such critical appraisal will imply the systematic assessment of the robustness of the evidence and will be the most powerful tool in the process of learning what levels of evidence sustain the current knowledge in a given topic.

We define critical appraisal as an evaluation process which determines the significance or worth of something by careful appraisal and study. Thus, the critical appraisal of information regarding a given public health issue will be embedded and follow the seven-step procedure outlined in the previous section, and will aim to assess whether such information qualifies as evidence and to what extent.

The expertise created in public health has provided us with multiple and powerful tools to approach the critical appraisal of information. Hence critical appraisal tools have been designed and are utilised for the assessment of a very wide range of documents reporting on findings from public health activities. Critical appraisal tools available for different types of public health activities (research papers, programme assessment, policies reviews and so on) will be presented, explained and their applicability demonstrated in detail in Chapter 4. However, the generic questioning exercise that an appraisal system will facilitate in evaluating both the quality and strength of findings from a public health review and the value of the search performed are described below (Guyatt and Drummond, 2002; Brownson *et al.*, 2003).

What are the results?

- Did the studies reviewed produce similar findings?
- What are the overall results of the review?
- How precise were the results?

Could a causal association be inferred from the available data?

- Are the results valid?
- Did the review explicitly address the public health question?
- Was the search for relevant studies detailed and exhaustive? Is it likely that important, relevant studies were missed?
- Were the primary studies of high methodological quality?
- Were the assessments of studies reproducible?

How can the results be applied to public health practice and interventions?

- How can the results be interpreted and applied to public health?
- Were all important public health outcomes considered?
- Are the benefits worth the costs and potential risks?

Chapter summary

In this chapter we started with the broad definition of EBPH as 'the conscientious explicit and judicious use of current best evidence in making decisions about the care of communities and populations in the domain of health protection, disease prevention, health maintenance and improvement' (Jenicek, 1997, pages 187–197) and we introduced you to the origins of modern EBPH from the emergence of EBM. We also discussed the key features of EBPH:

- conceptual plausibility;

- use of different types of evidence and translation of evidence into practical guidance for policy and practice.

Thus, EBPH is used:

- when scientific evidence must support decision making;

- to evaluate the effectiveness and cost benefits of public health programs;

- to implement new public health programs or interventions;

- when new policies must be established;

- to conduct literature reviews for grant projects.

Finally, we outlined the most important advantages of using EBPH in public health interventions as:

- it enables the decision-making processes to be based on scientific evidence and effective practices;

- it facilitates the retrieval of up-to-date and reliable information about what works and doesn't work for a given public health issue;

- it reassures on the efficiency of public health measures.

The chapter also included practical introductory guidance on how to gather information (with the inclusion of a suggested seven-step module) and what questions a critical appraisal on findings from public health research should include.

- Centre for Evidence Based Public Health Policy www.sphsu.mrc.ac.uk/
  Evidence/Evidence.html
  *This website is the virtual tool of the ESRC, responding to the growing demand for
  rational and effective policy interventions in public health. Both training activities
  and outputs of their research activities can be accessed there.*

- The Cochrane Collaboration www.cochrane.org
  *Unmissable portal to access to information on evidence in public health and in
  medicine.*

- London Health Observatory www.lho.org.uk
  *The LHO is an organisation devoted to monitoring health and health care in Lon-
  don through support to practitioners and information feed to policy makers. It is an
  essential website for those interested in learning how the health of the population is
  monitored in London.*

chapter 2

What are Sources of Evidence?

Amina Dilmohamed and Mahwish Hayee

Meeting the public health competences

Core area 2: Assessing the evidence of effectiveness of interventions, programmes and services to improve population health and wellbeing.

This chapter will help you to evidence the following competences for public health (Public Health Skills and Careers Framework):

- Level 6 (a) Understanding of how to search literature
- Level 6 (b) Knowledge of the principles of critical appraisal as applied to various studies, and its use in improving health and wellbeing
- Level 6 (c) Understanding of the levels of evidence and their importance for decision-making in own area of work
- Level 7 (b) Understanding of the hierarchy of evidence as it applies to services, programmes and interventions which impact on health and wellbeing.

This chapter will also assist you in demonstrating the following National Occupational Standard(s) for public health:

- Reflect on and develop your practice – (HSC33)
- Encourage innovation in your area of responsibility – (M&L C2)
- Facilitate the clinical audit process – (HI124)
- Search for clinical information and evidence according to an accepted methodology (HI125)
- Develop evidence-based clinical guidelines – (HI127).

This chapter will also be useful in demonstrating Standards 4c and 4e and 7 of the Public Health Practitioner Standards.

- Standard 4. Continually develop and improve own and others' practice in public health by:

    d. the application of evidence in improving own area of work
    e. objectively and constructively contributing to reviewing the effectiveness of own area of work.

- Standard 7. Assess the evidence of effective interventions and services to improve health and wellbeing – demonstrating:

    a. knowledge of the different types, sources and levels of evidence in own area of practice and how to access and use them
    b. the appraisal of published evidence and the identification of implications for own area of work practice.

Chapter overview

This chapter presents the sources of evidence applicable to public health. It also introduces the Cochrane Collaboration and provides a comprehensive guidance on database searching techniques. The purpose of this chapter is to identify and introduce the various sources of evidence. Public health evidence can be obtained from many sources but the important step is how to identify and determine the credible sources of evidence. It is important to note that there are several study designs and the quality of study varies. Studies need to adhere to the standard study design and methodology in order for it to hold credence. For novices in the field of public health it is important to find appropriate evidence and to understand how this should be used in public health practice.

What this chapter intends to do is give you step-by-step guidance in searching the public health literature. What has become hard, especially for those new to the field of public health, is to find appropriate evidence and then to understand how it should be used in public health practice. However, as a researcher it must be understood that there are many sources of evidence and all have to be taken into consideration and information should be collected from all sources. Their scientific robustness should be judged and then they should be added to the general pool of knowledge.

This chapter will help you to meet the following competences for public health in understanding the different sources of evidence:

- To understand what is meant by sources of evidence
- To understand the Cochrane Collaboration
- An introduction of different quantitative research designs
- To acquire skills of database search.

Exercises in this chapter will focus on:

- recognising the place of the different sources of evidence in the hierarchy of evidence;
- understanding how studies are searched from the Cochrane Collaboration and what important components are needed to read about a paper;
- developing a search strategy when looking for public health evidence.

Public health practitioners and specialists are regularly required to find sources of evidence and use it in their practice, in public health projects, public health evaluations or to inform policy. In order to help you to identify ways to find evidence more effectively, in this chapter the key steps of the process will be explored. A number of useful steps that need to be used at each stage are introduced and discussed here. By reading this chapter you will understand the different steps in searching for public health literature and will be able to link it with other chapters in this book.

Steps in searching public health literature

In the first chapter of this book you were introduced to evidence-based public health and the different ways it can be utilised to look for evidence. In this chapter we will look at what steps are taken for searching for public health literature specifically. We will also discuss the credible sources for looking for public health research. After finding suitable sources, a public health practitioner or specialist should be able to use appropriate search terms and we will discuss these here in detail.

The first step is to look for the public health problem that you are going to solve. Once this is established you need to clearly define your question. Then you need to look for information sources. These are the sources that you intend to look in to do your research. Then you need to use the search strategy explained in this chapter in order to come up with key terms that you will use in your search.

The next step is to conduct the search. Your search will give you many results but you will have to use your own judgement to select documents that are relevant to your research for reviewing. You need to first read the titles of all the identified articles and also the abstracts. Once you have read these you need to select the ones relevant to your research question and document them or keep them in a safe place for reviewing. Remember to remove titles and abstracts that are duplicates or that are not relevant to your research. In this step the application of inclusion/exclusion criteria is very helpful. The criteria specify which studies are to be included and excluded in your research process. Whenever you decide these criteria, always try to justify your choice by thinking it through in detail. These will define the studies that the search strategy is attempting to locate. If you have difficulty in understanding what these are, you can think of it as being similar to the process by which authors of primary research define the samples and populations that they intend to study and draw conclusions about. This will help you to make sure you include what you think is relevant and exclude what you think may not be relevant to your research. Finally read and summarise all the information that you have collected for your research (Brownson *et al.*, 2003, page 128).

Selection of information sources

In Chapter 1 you would have clearly understood how you can determine or define a public health question using a PICO (Patient, Intervention, Comparator, and Outcome) framework. There are activities in Chapter 1 that can be done to further understand this concept.

Now we will talk about the different information sources.

- Systematic reviews and meta-analyses
- Observational studies
- Practice guidelines
- Best practices.

Systematic reviews and meta-analyses

A systematic review is the critical assessment and evaluation of research that attempts to address a focused question using methods designed to reduce the likelihood of bias. Whenever a systematic review is conducted, explicit methods are used to locate primary studies, and explicit criteria are used to assess their quality. Following these specified criteria improves the credibility of the study.

After discussing the systematic review we will talk about the meta-analysis. This is an overview that incorporates a quantitative strategy for combining the results of several studies into a single pooled or summary estimate. Basically, a meta-analysis will thoroughly examine a number of valid studies on a topic and combine the results using accepted statistical methodology as if they were from one large study. In public health practice some practitioners consider meta-analysis to be superior to a systematic review, because part of the methodology includes critical appraisal of the selected randomised controlled trials and a quantitative analysis of pooling of data is carried out (Brownson *et al.*, 2003).

Randomised controlled clinical trials are carefully planned projects that study the effect of a therapy on real patients. They include methodologies that reduce the potential for bias (randomisation and blinding) and that allow for comparison between intervention groups and control groups (no intervention). Individuals are randomly allocated to a control group and a group who receive a specific intervention. Otherwise the two groups are identical for any significant variables. They are followed up for specific end points.

Observational studies

Broadly speaking, two types of observational studies are discussed here: cohort studies and case–control studies. In cohort studies groups of people are selected on the basis of their exposure to a particular agent and followed up for specific outcomes. Cohort studies take a large population and follow patients who have a specific condition or receive a particular treatment over time and compare them with another group that has not been affected by the condition or treatment being studied. Cohort studies are observational and not as reliable as randomised controlled studies, since the two groups may differ in ways other than in the variable under study.

The other type of observational study is a case–control study. In this study design patients who already have a specific condition are compared with people who do not. They often rely on medical records and patient recall for data collection. These types of studies are often less reliable than randomised controlled trials and cohort studies because showing a statistical relationship does not mean that one factor necessarily caused the other.

Practice guidelines

Simply stated, practice guidelines are systematically developed statements to assist practitioner and patient decisions about appropriate health care for specific clinical circumstances. These may have been developed by government agencies, institutions or by the convening of expert panels. Public health specialists in the UK may refer to practice guidelines produced by National Institute for Health and Clinical Excellence (NICE), the Faculty of Public Health or Department of Health.

Best practices

There is no universally accepted definition of best practice. For our own understanding we can consider public health programmes, interventions and policies that through experience have been evaluated, shown to be successful and have the potential to be adapted and transformed by others working in the same field to be examples of best practice. As public health practitioner you need to look for the following characteristics to ascertain whether these are examples of best practice and not any other research design:

- Lacks rigorous evaluation of a systematic review or meta-analysis

- Applied across a variety of public health areas

- Vary widely in scope, methods, and quality

- Expert opinion to systematic methods

- Some are very influential.

ACTIVITY 2.1

Figure 2.1 is a diagrammatic guide to levels of evidence. As a public health specialist or practitioner you should be able to place the different study types according to their hierarchy. Do this exercise so you can remember where the studies should be placed.

If you can't do it, you will find this pyramid in Chapter 9 where you will learn how the studies are placed. Once you have seen that come back to fill this in.

Sources of credible evidence

One problem with public health is that the resources do not tend to be all in one (or even three or four places), as they are in medicine. Therefore, public health practitioners and specialists should know about credible sources for looking for evidence. In this chapter we have discussed some important sources of evidence; make sure you familiarise yourself with these.

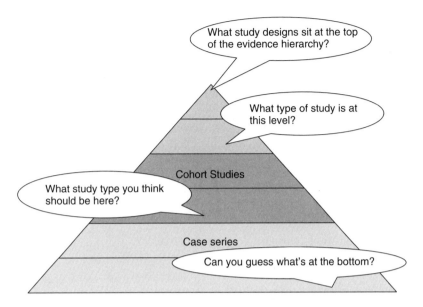

Figure 2.1

The Cochrane Collaboration

First we will discuss the Cochrane Collaboration, how it was started and what it is used for. The Cochrane Collaboration was founded in 1993 under the leadership of Iain Chalmers. It was developed in response to Archie Cochrane's call for up-to-date, systematic reviews of all relevant randomised controlled trials of health care. The Research and Development Programme was initiated to support the United Kingdom's National Health Service. Funds were provided to establish a 'Cochrane Centre', to collaborate with others, in the UK and elsewhere, to facilitate systematic reviews of randomised controlled trials across all areas of health care.

The benefits of the Cochrane Library

The Cochrane Library is a vast source of evidence bringing together international research on the effectiveness of health care treatments and interventions. It has an extensive research reservoir of over 6000 Cochrane systematic reviews and over 650 000 other records, covering clinical trials, methods, technology and economic evaluations. The library ensures that the best research evidence with clinical expertise and patient values is maintained. The entire source is reliable because they adhere to a strict methodology to ensure that Cochrane reviews are comprehensive, thus minimising bias. Furthermore, the Cochrane reviews are updated monthly, ensuring that treatment decisions can be based on the most up-to-date, reliable evidence. More importantly for research trainees or students, it has a comprehensive and flexible viewing and searching functionality using Medical Subject Heading (MeSH).

MeSH Search is based on the National Library of Medicine's controlled vocabulary thesaurus of medical subject headings. It includes both an alphabetical and hierarchical listing of related sets that allow you to browse lists for specific terms. The MeSH search feature can be accessed by clicking on the MeSH search link on the navigation bar on the Cochrane Advanced page or the MeSH search link in the search box on the Cochrane Library homepage.

The Cochrane Library is a collection of evidence-based medicine databases which include systematic reviews that are updated monthly. There are several databases in the Cochrane Library collection:

- The Cochrane Database of Systematic Reviews (Cochrane Reviews)
- The Cochrane Database of Abstracts of Reviews of Effects (other reviews)
- The Cochrane Central Register of Controlled Trials (clinical trials)
- The Cochrane Methodology Register (methods studies)
- Health Technology Assessment Database (technology assessments)
- NHS Economic Evaluation Database (economic evaluations).

It is essential that after reading this chapter you become familiar with the Cochrane Collaboration's work and database and understand that it is an important and reliable source of evidence base in public health. Cochrane Reviews is now the 'gold standard' for systematic reviews in the following key publications:

- *The Lancet*
- *New England Journal of Medicine*
- *British Medical Journal*
- *Journal of the American Medical Association*

and routinely appears in these as well as in specialised medical journals.

ACTIVITY 2.2 HOW TO SEARCH THE COCHRANE LIBRARY AND WHAT TO LOOK AT IN A PAPER

Search the Cochrane Library for review abstracts on inhaler therapy for asthma. How many reviews do you find? Select one of the reviews and summarise the 'Main Results' and 'Reviewers' Conclusions'.

Example: what might happen if you undertake the task in Activity 2.2

The Cochrane Library was searched and five abstracts were retrieved for studies that looked at the role of a single inhaler in asthma therapy. One article was selected and the review was retrieved. The intervention reviewed combination formoterol and budesonide as maintenance and reliever therapy versus inhaled steroid maintenance for chronic asthma in adults and children.

Five studies on 5378 adults compared single inhaler therapy with current best practice, and did not show a significant reduction in participants with exacerbations causing hospitalisation (Peto odds ratio (OR) 0.59; 95% confidence interval (95% CI) 0.24 to 1.45) or treated with oral steroids (OR 0.83; 95% CI 0.66 to 1.03). Three of these studies on 4281 adults did not show a significant reduction in time to first severe exacerbation needing medical intervention (hazard ratio (HR) 0.96; 95% CI 0.85 to 1.07). These trials demonstrated a reduction in the mean total daily dose of inhaled corticosteroids with single inhaler therapy (mean reduction ranged from 107 to 267 micrograms/day, but the trial results were not combined due to heterogeneity). The full results from four further studies on 4600 adults comparing single inhaler therapy with current best practice are awaited.

Three studies including 4209 adults compared single inhaler therapy with higher dose budesonide maintenance and terbutaline for symptom relief. No significant reduction was found with single inhaler therapy in the risk of patients suffering an asthma exacerbation leading to hospitalisation (Peto OR 0.56; 95% CI 0.28 to 1.09), but fewer patients on single inhaler therapy needed a course of oral corticosteroids (OR 0.54; 95% CI 0.45 to 0.64). These results translate into an 11-month number needed to treat of 14 (95% CI 12 to 18) to prevent one patient being treated with oral corticosteroids for an exacerbation. The run-in for these studies involved withdrawal of long-acting beta2-agonists, and patients were recruited who were symptomatic during run-in.

One study included children (N = 224), in which single inhaler therapy was compared to higher dose budesonide. There was a significant reduction in participants who needed an increase in their inhaled steroids with single inhaler therapy, but there were only two hospitalisations for asthma and no separate data on courses of oral corticosteroids. Fewer inhaled and oral corticosteroids were used in the single inhaler therapy group and the annual height gain was also 1 cm greater in the single inhaler therapy group (95% CI 0.3 to 1.7 cm).

There was no significant difference found in fatal or non-fatal serious adverse events for any of the comparisons.

The author's conclusion is that single inhaler therapy can reduce the risk of asthma exacerbations needing oral corticosteroids in comparison with fixed dose maintenance inhaled corticosteroids. Guidelines and common best practice suggest the addition of regular long-acting beta2-agonist to inhaled corticosteroids for uncontrolled asthma, and single inhaler therapy has not been demonstrated to significantly reduce exacerbations in comparison with current best practice, although results of five large trials are awaiting full publication. Single inhaler therapy is not currently licensed for children under 18 years of age in the UK.

PubMed

PubMed is another important search engine for searching literature. It contains all citations from the medical literature dating back from 1953. It is also very up to date as it is linked directly to publishers and the home pages of the journals. It is worthwhile noting that MEDLINE is hosted on PubMed.

Bibliographic database sources

When you start your research, make sure you look at the Cochrane Collaboration and PubMed but this does not mean that you should end your search here. There are also other databases. In the later part of the chapter we will be talking about the different databases that can be used for your literature search. These will be briefly discussed here so that you can become familiar with the names.

MEDLINE

Produced by the National Library of Medicine, MEDLINE provides extensive coverage of the world's biomedical journal literature with a broad coverage which includes basic biomedical research and the clinical sciences, since 1966.

Embase (The excerpta medica database)

Produced by Elsevier Science, Embase is a major biomedical and pharmaceutical database indexing over 3500 international journals. It is current and the most frequently used – approximately 375 000 records are added annually.

CINAHL

This is the major bibliographic database for English language journals in nursing and allied health fields. Around 1200 journals are selected and comprehensively indexed. Publications of the American Nurses' Association and the National League for Nursing are included, as well as books in nursing and allied health.

PsycINFO

This covers the professional and academic literature in psychology and related disciplines. Coverage is worldwide references and abstracts to over 1300 journals and dissertations in more than 30 languages; 5000 references are added a month and it promises that nearly 100 000 records will be added every year.

DARE (Database of Abstracts of Reviews of Effectiveness)

High-quality systematic reviews, also part of evidence-based medicine.

Trip Database

Searches over 75 sites for medical information with direct hyperlink access to the largest collection of 'evidence base' material on the web, including premier journals (e.g. *BMJ, JAMA*) which do not have free access.

CenterWatch clinical trials listing services

The information source for the clinical trials industry contains information on clinical research listing >41 000 active industry and government sponsored clinical trials, as well as new drug therapies in research approved by the FDA. The site is open to patients interested in participating in clinical trials and for research professionals.

Government reports

These can be accessed on the internet via whichever government department has commissioned the report. The Department of Health has many reports about public health policies.

Dissertation theses

The 'Index to Theses' database is a comprehensive listing of theses with abstracts accepted for higher degrees by universities in Great Britain and Ireland since 1716. It can be accessed via the 'E-resources via Search it' pages on the Library and Information Service website. Full texts for theses can sometimes be obtained from the British Library EThOS Service.

British Library EThOS (Electronic Theses Online Service)

This is a new service from the British Library. Digitised copies of theses are available to download from participating universities. All users need to register and login before they can use the service. A thesis that has not yet been digitised can be ordered via Library and Information Service and the British Library will digitise it and make it available for download.

National Institute for Health and Clinical Excellence (NICE)

NICE is the independent organisation responsible for providing national guidance on the promotion of good health and the prevention and treatment of ill health. NICE produces clinical guidance in three areas:

- Public health – promotion of good health and prevention of ill health

- Health technologies – the use of new and existing medicine, treatments and procedures

- Clinical practice – appropriate treatment of people with specific diseases within the NHS.

Search techniques

Now you are clear about what search engines to use when you search for literature one thing that you need to learn are the different search techniques that are available. These include:

- Keywords

- Boolean searching

- Combining words

- Phrase searching

- Truncation/wildcard searching

- Focusing a search

- List of databases

- Keeping a record of your searches.

Keywords

This is very important and you should think very carefully about the keywords you select to define your search topic. Spend some time selecting the keywords and think about the important terms included in your topic area. What you come up with will be based on personal choice and you will find that two research studies done on the same topic do not necessarily use the same terms. Also pay attention to the following:

- Synonyms – these are different words with the same meaning (e.g. cancer and neoplasm)

- Acronyms – this is where your keywords can be condensed into a set of capital letters (e.g. CHD cardiovascular disease). Use both the full term and the acronym when searching

- Alternative spellings – remember to try UK and US spellings, for example paediatric and pediatric

- Try to be broad as well as specific so that you get the right information

- Look at ways to link your keywords. Do you want records that contain all of your keywords or are some alternatives; do you want to relate two words so that they are near each other; can you focus your search by excluding words which might appear with other words you are searching for but in a different context?

- Many databases provide a thesaurus of keywords, which is used to classify the work held in the database. Use this helpful tool if possible, as it provides consistency when searching.

It is also helpful to think about how the terms could be linked together (e.g. a search on the government public health policy may need to be combined with UK).

Boolean searching

Boolean operators allow you to join terms together, widen a search or exclude terms from your search results. This means you can be more precise in locating your information. Not all search tools support Boolean searching.

- AND – using this narrows your search by combining words. The results found must contain all the words which you have joined by using AND.

- OR – using this broadens your search to include resources which contain any or all of the terms connected by OR.

- NOT or AND NOT – narrows your search by excluding a term.

Combining words

As well as using the boolean operators (explained above) to combine words, there are other ways of connecting search terms to narrow down your results. This is a highly effective way of making your results more specific and relevant and most databases do offer this. So look for it whenever you are using a search engine.

Phrase searching

This is used when an extract phrase or sentence is being looked for. This can be very useful when a search is being made for an exact title or quotation. It can be used in three ways in search tools. The most common is to use speech marks, for example "pulmonary tuberculosis"; this will then find studies that have used the exact phrase. In other search tools you may have to use (brackets) or single quote marks, for example 'whooping cough'.

Truncation/wildcard searching

These search techniques retrieve information on similar words by replacing part of the word with a symbol, usually a * or ? However, different databases use different symbols, so check what is used.

- In truncation, the end of the word is replaced. For example physiother* will retrieve physiotherapy, physiotherapeutic, physiotherapist and so on.

- In wildcard searching, letters from inside the word are replaced. For example m*n with retrieve the terms man and men.

Example: search techniques

You have been tasked to look at whether aspirin works in the treatment of heart attack. You may choose MEDLINE. To do this, a search strategy will usually comprise both indexing terms (if the database has a thesaurus or controlled vocabulary) and 'free text' terms and synonyms (from the database record's title and abstract) to ensure that as many relevant papers are retrieved as possible. For example, when searching MEDLINE for studies about myocardial infarction, the free text term 'heart attack' should be used as well as the MeSH term 'myocardial infarction'. Identifying appropriate indexing terms can be done by searching for key papers and checking how they have been indexed, as well as by scanning the thesaurus for relevant terms.

Another important thing to remember in this search is when selecting free text terms to use in the strategy it is important to take account of alternative spellings (including US and British English variants), abbreviations, synonyms, geographical variation, and changes in terminology over time. Sometimes it can also be useful to search for common mis-spellings, for example 'asprin' when you want to retrieve studies of aspirin.

This shows you that you need to be careful about your search terms and make sure you do them appropriately.

Focusing a search/setting limitations

This is very important and you should carefully think about how to do this. There are many ways to focus your search and all search tools offer different techniques. Check the help facilities if the options are not immediately obvious. Some of the ways of limiting your search are as follows:

- Date – what date you want to start and till when. Most commonly the month and year of start and the month and year you want to look at is included in this.

- Language – do you want the search to be only in English or you want to include other languages? Whatever you decide specify it.

- Place – what country? Specify if you want to just include research from UK or you want to add other countries such as USA or Australia, for example.

- Publication type – what types of publication or documentation do you wish to include. This is also sometimes called the range.

- Age groups – what age group? Only children 1–10 years or adults 30–50 years?

- Gender – do you want to include both males and females?

- Type of material – you may wish to find only randomised controlled trials.

Make a list of sources/databases

It is up to you to decide on your list and depending on the availability of resources/ sources, these may be print-based or computer-based. In this chapter most of the commonly used databases are listed so you can use them.

Keep a record of your searches

An essential part of literature searching is keeping accurate, consistent and correct records. These should include the years of every print-based and electronic database searched, and the terms used.

Also, useful references should be recorded from print-based sources or marked and downloaded from electronic databases. This will help in making the reference list. Also, you should be familiar with writing the citation.

How to assess different sources of evidence

When you have identified the relevant literature you need to assess it for its quality. We have introduced some basic steps you need to take to review the paper. In other sections of the book you will be able to understand the detailed way you can do this. Briefly, there are three broad questions to consider before reviewing a paper:

1. Is the study valid?

2. Is the study reliable?

3. Will the study results help locally?

(Public Health Resource Unit, 2010)

Assessing evidence is not an easy task and therefore for you to be able to answer the questions suggested by the Public Health Resource Unit, you need to be clear about what the questions mean. I have tried to explain them in simple terms.

1. Validity in simple words means closeness to the truth (Greenhalgh, 2006). A valid measure is the one which measures what it is suppose to measure. For example, when estimating alcohol consumption, valid answers are unlikely to be obtained to the question 'how much do you drink?' Many subjects will understate their true consumption, although some boastful ones may exaggerate (Crombie, 2007).

2. Reliability is the repeatability of the tests. As an example, in theory the height of an adult should be reliably measured, as it varies only slightly throughout the day. Good high-quality studies do discuss how reliability was assessed (Crombie, 2007).

3. Look at the topic as well as the finding of the study and judge by asking yourself the question whether the finding of the study will help locally in your practice.

Were the patients studied similar to the ones you come across and were the conditions in which the study was carried out similar to local circumstances?

Steps to be followed

1. Start with a clear focused question.

2. Look for a systematic review from Cochrane Collaboration or MEDLINE.

3. If you find it, read it and think and judge by simple common sense the validity and reliability of the study as mentioned earlier.

4. If you think it is has answered the treatment or intervention question you are seeking then read the results section, a bit of the discussion, conclusion and the author's summary to find the answer.

5. If you cannot find a systematic review, look for a randomised controlled trial from the Cochrane Collaborations library of randomised controlled trials, MEDLINE or some other database.

6. If you cannot find randomised controlled trials or have been able to find only one then look for other study types and follow the same steps as before. Try locating at least 3 to 5 studies for a particular treatment and place the results together.

7. In the following tables studies have been further discussed and explanation of each study type has been given in detail so that researchers can easily understand what type of study they are looking at.

Case study 2.1: Steps that need to taken to search for evidence

A student doctor is researching the attitudes of different staff to handwashing. She first searches the literature to focus the scope of the original question. Although the literature on handwashing is vast, she needs to discover whether published research has been conducted, specifically in obstetrics and gynaecology settings. Has anyone researched the topic specifically in a delivery suite? 'Handwashing' has many more definitions than she had envisaged. Does handwashing include the use of a hand rub? Does it constitute use of water only? What is the minimum duration of the procedure before it is classed as 'handwashing'? The literature search enables her to explore different definitions of her main concepts.

Are there validated instruments to measure attitudes to handwashing (or towards routine hospital hygiene)? The literature review may inform selection of appropriate outcomes – those employed in previous studies or those considered appropriate by the relevant clinical community. Will she focus singly on attitudes or will she investigate knowledge and/or behaviour? She put the search term 'handwashing' in PubMed. The search revealed 1213 titles and abstracts using the word handwashing. After reading the titles and abstracts she shortlisted 800 articles. Then she applied the inclusion and exclusion criteria set by her for this study. She ended up with 55 articles that were used in the review.

ACTIVITY 2.3

After reading Case study 2.1:

1. What structured process needs to be used before searching the literature?
2. Can you identify the keywords used in this case study?
3. Do you think that the student doctor has used appropriate search techniques for this review?

Spend a few minutes thinking about these questions.

Chapter summary

In this chapter we started with the broad discussion about the different sources of evidence in public health. Then we discussed the steps a public health specialist or practitioner needs to take to look for appropriate sources for evidence. We introduced the different information resources and the different study designs to guide the reader. Then we looked at the subject-appropriate databases, mainly the Cochrane Collaboration and PubMed. We also introduced the reader to other sources of evidence which they can consult to find public health evidence. We have also discussed how a search strategy needs to be constructed and have detailed all the steps that need to be taken.

- The Cochrane Collaboration www.cochrane.org
  A rich source of systematic reviews. Established in 1993, it is an international net-work of people helping health care providers, policy makers, patients, their advocates and carers; it makes well-informed decisions about human health care by preparing, updating and promoting the accessibility of Cochrane Reviews – over 4000 so far, published online in the Cochrane Library.

- Centre for Evidence Based Public Health Policy www.sphsu.mrc.ac.uk/ Evidence/Evidence.html
  This website is the virtual tool of the ESRC responding to the growing demand for rational and effective policy interventions in public health.

- Critical Appraisal Skills Programme www.phru.nhs.uk/casp/casp.htm
  CASP aims to enable individuals to develop the skills to find and make sense of research evidence, helping them to put knowledge into practice. www.phru.nhs.uk/ casp/casp.htm

- PubMed www.ncbi.nlm.nih.gov/pubmed
  PubMed comprises over 20 million citations for biomedical literature from MEDLINE, life science journals and online books which include the fields of medi-cine, nursing, dentistry, veterinary medicine, the health care system and preclinical sciences. PubMed also provides access to additional relevant websites and links to the other National Center for Biotechnology Information (NCBI) molecular biology resources.

chapter 3

Making Sense of the Evidential Hierarchy Used to Judge Research Evidence

Nena Foster

Meeting the public health competences

Core area 2: Assessing the evidence of effectiveness of interventions, programmes and services to improve population health and wellbeing.

This chapter will help you to evidence the following competences for public health (Public Health Skills and Careers Framework):

- Level 6 (1) Frame a question to be used as the basis for reviewing literature in relation to evidence on a specific issue
- Level 6 (2) Identify, collect and collate the evidence that is needed to answer a question on a specific issue
- Level 6 (3) Synthesise, appraise and summarise evidence on a specific issue
- Level 6 (4) Communicate findings of the appraisal of evidence on a specific issue
- Level 6 (5) Apply evidence within own area of work
- Level 6(c) Understand the levels of evidence and their importance for decision-making in own areas of work
- Level 7 (1) Critically appraise and summarise evidence from a range of sources
- Level 7 (2) Formulate recommendations for change on the basis of critically appraised evidence
- Level 7 (b) Understanding the hierarchy of evidence as it applies to services, programmes and interventions which impact on health and wellbeing
- Level 8 (1) Make and influence decisions based on evidence of effectiveness.

This chapter will also assist you in demonstrating the following National Occupational Standard(s) for public health:

- Assess the evidence and impact of health and health care interventions, programmes and services and apply the assessments to practice – (PHS07)
- Improve the quality of health and health care interventions and services through audit and evaluation – (PHS08)
- Support and challenge workers on specific aspects of their practice – (CJF309).

This chapter will also be useful in demonstrating Standards 4c and 4e and 7 of the Public Health Practitioner Standards.

- Standard 4. Continually develop and improve own and others' practice in public health by:

  d. the application of evidence in improving own area of work

e. objectively and constructively contributing to reviewing the effectiveness of own area of work.

- Standard 7. Assess the evidence of effective interventions and services to improve health and wellbeing – demonstrating:

    a. knowledge of the different types, sources and levels of evidence in own area of practice and how to access and use them
    b. the appraisal of published evidence and the identification of implications for own area of work practice.

Chapter overview

In the previous chapters we have addressed the need for and nature of 'evidence' as relevant to changing and informing best practices to promote health and wellbeing within public health. This chapter sets out to examine the nature and strength of research evidence in more detail. As we have seen, finding the best evidence can often be a difficult task, as the sheer amount of information available can be overwhelming, and the information available can vary in quality. When faced with large amounts of information, some of which may present contradictory or inconclusive results, the task of finding the best or strongest available evidence seems an onerous one, albeit necessary, particularly when life/death or better/worse health depends upon it.

In this chapter we explore the relationship between a study's research design and the level or strength of research evidence provided by these designs that can be utilised to make the best or most informed decisions about the effectiveness of public health interventions, programmes and services. First, we will examine the ability of various research designs to address different types of research questions before examining the hierarchical ranking system, known as the 'evidential hierarchy' which is utilised or order or rank particular research designs. Next, the chapter will examine the various research designs and their corresponding methodological principles in detail before providing some examples activities. Finally, the chapter will discuss the limitations of the hierarchy in terms of addressing research quality beyond the use of a specific research design.

Exercises in this chapter will focus on:

- exploring different types of evidence;
- appreciating and understanding the evidential hierarchy;
- considering alternatives to the evidential hierarchy.

After reading this chapter you will be able to:

- appreciate the strengths and weaknesses of different types of evidence and their potential use in improving population health and wellbeing;
- understand what is meant by the evidential hierarchy;
- appreciate the ability of different research designs to answer specific research questions;
- understand different study designs and appreciate the level of evidence they might provide.

One design does not fit all research queries

When we research we have a specific research question in mind, and this research question is designed to investigate a particular research problem. In general, research queries can be answered qualitatively or quantitatively, and occasionally, using both quantitative and qualitative methods may be necessary. For example, you may want to know what evidence is available about the effectiveness of harm reduction strategies for reducing the incidence of TB infection among injecting drug users, which would require pooling existing research evidence, or you may want to investigate patient perceptions of community-facilitated aged care services, which would involve collect your own data. As you can imagine, there are many types of research queries and unsurprisingly, different methodological approaches that are useful and appropriate to address these different queries.

Not only are some research designs better suited to addressing certain types of research questions, as we will see later in the chapter, but it is also important to note that employing a particular research design also means adhering to a set of methodological principles, or guidelines prescribed by the appropriated research design. Adherence to these guidelines is integral to distinguishing the research design and, as addressed in this chapter, integral to the ranking or the level evidence provided by the study. The rest of this chapter is devoted to exploring in detail the various levels and types of research evidence.

ACTIVITY 3.1

There are various types and sources of information that we use in everyday life that we use to inform our decisions and opinions. Take a look at the sources of information below and rank these in order or from most reliable (1) to least reliable (8). Reflect on your criteria for ranking these information sources.

- Local news/newspapers
- National news/newspapers
- Your own views or judgements
- Views or judgements of those you deem to be wise or respected
- Local government information
- National government information
- Information from the private or business sector report
- Internet websites or blogs

   Comment: You probably found it easy to distinguish between the reliability of your own views or judgements and the views or judgements of those you respect and local or national newspapers. Where you positioned local government or national government information will depend on your view of government as a source of information. The same will be true for internet websites or blogs. Given the complexity of the types and sources of public health information it is crucial that we develop a way of distinguishing reliable and less reliable information and develop a framework for ranking levels and types of evidence.

Guidelines for finding quality evidence

Researchers and public health practitioners are often faced with finding the proof or evidence that a particular programme, treatment or intervention has been effective in improving health and/or wellbeing. Likewise, they are charged with the task as researchers of designing suitably effective programmes or interventions to address a public health problem or concern. In order to undertake both of these tasks, it is important to find, review as well as create the most reliable or best information to inform the next steps, whether this is making policy recommendations or implementing a particular programme.

Finding the best proof or evidence may seem like finding a needle in a haystack, considering the sheer amount of information available, and perhaps this would be the case if there were no framework or guidance to help locate higher or better evidence. Thus, in order to help select which information is most reliable or likely to be the most reliable in terms of providing reliable evidence, the evidential hierarchy serves as a starting point for finding reliable information. Within this hierarchy, research designs which are said to produce the highest level or the most reliable evidence are ranked higher than other types of evidence.

The framework or guidelines provided by this hierarchy not only serve as a guide to the level or strength of evidence provided by different types of research studies, but also tell us a bit about the likelihood of bias in the research. Bias refers to the occurrence or the potential for error in research, which is likely to impact on or provide incorrect research results; these are instances which research and researchers seek to mitigate or minimise, particularly in quantitative research.

In order to understand how the various research designs correspond to the level of evidence provided and its ability to minimise bias, we first must explore the origins of the evidential hierarchy and briefly address the various types of research evidence ordered within this framework.

Before examining the levels of evidence in detail, we will examine the history and structure of the evidential hierarchy, a system of ranking evidence. The evidential hierarchy as a ranking system for research evidence originated and continues to be used in biomedical and clinical research. This hierarchy has since been taken up and used by public health researchers, although its significance as a mechanism for accurately judging the quality of research evidence has been the subject of debate.

Origins and structure of the hierarchy

As discussed above, the framework used to rank research evidence is known as the 'hierarchy of evidence' or the 'evidential hierarchy', and the framework utilises a hierarchical system divided into several levels. Such a system was first proposed by Campbell and Stanley (1963) and popularised in the late 1970s in connection with the evidence-based medicine movement. This resulted in a usable framework developed by the Canadian Taskforce on the Periodic Health Examination (1979). While born from a clinical research tradition, this framework utilises commonly used clinical research designs, many of which are relevant to and widely used in public health research.

In particular, as discussed above, public health practitioners and researchers are faced with judging the effectiveness of an intervention, often a vital part of the processes of decision making within public health (i.e. whether or not to implement a particular intervention or strategy within a particular population), and there are a limited number of study designs which are capable of measuring or indicating levels of effectiveness. And in order to gauge or accurately measure effectiveness of a particular intervention we must be certain that the observed results are a product of the intervention efforts, rather than something external to the research or luck. Accordingly, the best level of evidence designed to answer questions related to effectiveness utilise an experimental design, and the hierarchical ranking system recognises and values this particular design's principles which ensure that once the research has been conducted, the researcher can comment with a fair amount of certainty on the intervention's ability to deliver the particular results. Thus, the commonly used and clinically influenced study designs often utilised in public health research are ranked or graded into levels based on their ability to produce more certain results, which is done to minimise the occurrence of the likelihood of bias (Rychetnik et al., 2002).

There are several ways to minimise the likelihood of bias occurring in research, which as indicated above is important for all quantitative research designs. An interventional study design means that there is a group which receives the intervention (experimental group) and a group that does not receive the intervention (control group). Often an interventional study design employs both random allocation of participants to the experimental and control groups and tests each group before and after (pre and post tests) to examine whether or not the intervention has had an impact on the outcome observed (Neuman, 2006). This type of experimental study design is utilised in a number of research disciplines, including medicine and public health. An experimental design that involves the random allocation of participation further decreases the likelihood of biased study results in order to provide true measures of intervention effectiveness; however, the ranking of the research alone is not a sure indication of likely bias in reported research, as there is evidence that there are as likely to be biases in the evidence produced by higher ranking designs as there are in lower ranked designs. This research design alone is not an indicator of bias in published research findings (Borgerson, 2009).

Due to the specificity of the experimental and interventional research design aimed at minimising bias, these study designs occupy a higher position in the research hierarchy than those designs that are less able or less concerned with minimising bias. When well designed, these studies produce more reliable evidence in terms of the effectiveness of interventions, than any other study design. Table 3.1 illustrates this hierarchical relationship between research designs, ranking the reliability of evidence provided by each. As a result of its position at the top or near the top, depending on which hierarchy is utilised, a randomised controlled trial (RCT) provides the best level of evidence of effectiveness in terms of a single empirical study. The strength of evidence from a single RCT is said to multiply, when evidence is pooled from several interventions, thereby positioning research designs which synthesise and/or re-analyse data from several RCTs at the top of the hierarchy. Thus, systematic reviews or meta-analyses, which we will explore in more detail, are said to provide the highest level of evidence in terms of public health interventions (Centre for Reviews and Dissemination, 2009).

Table 3.1 Levels of evidence

Level	Description of evidence
I–1	Systematic review or meta-analyses of two or more RCTs
I–2	Randomised controlled trial
II–1	Cohort study
II–2	Case–control study
II–3	Cross-sectional study
II–4	Case-series study
III	Evidence from well-designed non-experimental studies (i.e. descriptive studies quantitative studies, qualitative studies)
IV	Expert opinion, clinical evidence, evidence from committee reports
V	Someone once told me . . . or evidence from peers/colleagues

Source: Adapted from Gillam *et al.* (2007, page 62) and Petticrew and Roberts (2003, page 527).

As illustrated in Table 3.1, evidence generated from the various types of research designs is ranked into levels based on the research design's ability to produce scientifically verifiable and less biased findings. Going down the hierarchy the strength of the evidence changes, becoming less reliable. As you will see, in terms of single empirical studies, experimental or quasi-experimental designs top the ranking system. As explained above, experimental and quasi-experimental designs involve the allocation of participants or 'subjects' to control and intervention groups for the purpose of comparing the outcome of receiving the intervention or treatment to the group that does not receive treatment (control group), thus relying on the scientific principles. Research designs such as RCTs (Level I–2 in Table 3.1) employ a classical experimental design and are said to provide the highest level of evidence, indicated by their position near the top of the hierarchy, while non-experimental designs are placed nearer the bottom (Centre for Reviews and Dissemination, 2009).

Next, we explore each of these levels in more detail in order to gain better insight into the methodological principles that correspond to the various study designs and the justification for the rank or position of the various designs in the hierarchy.

Exploring the levels of the hierarchy

Here we will explore the various levels of the framework as outlined in Table 3.1. This section provides an account of the types of study designs and the level of unbiased or bias-minimised evidence which these studies provide, according to the evidential hierarchy. As mentioned earlier in the chapter, this system is structured according to the design's ability to reduce or minimise bias, which skews research results and impacts on the quality and legitimacy of the evidence produced. While this framework provides a useful tool for weighting biases, it only provides a guide rather than a true indication of research quality. We will explore in more detail in Chapter 4 ways to examine, in-depth, research quality.

There are several research designs which provide the same level of evidence according to the hierarchy. For example, both systematic reviews and RCTs are assigned to Level I, but, as you will notice above, even within the levels there is a hierarchical ranking. This is illustrated best by Level II, as there are four different experimental research designs which provide the same level of evidence and some of these designs provide more reliable evidence than others. As shown above, a cohort study design is better equipped to produce less biased findings than a case serried design. Next, we will explore these various study designs and hopefully it will become clear why certain designs occupy certain positions on the hierarchy above or below other types of designs.

Level I–1: Systematic review and/or meta-analyses

While there are two research designs that provide highly reliable or Level I evidence, as noted above, Level I is split into two tiers, with the top tier occupied by synthesis research designs (pooling research evidence from multiple research studies). A single RCT is said to provide the highest level of evidence that can be provided by a single research study; however, the top of the hierarchy is reserved for research designs that pool and filter information from several individual studies (Sackett *et al.*, 2000). These processes are important to this study design, as it involves pooling, appraising and re-analysing the findings from two or more studies, often RCTs; however, depending on the subject areas and the available information, studies using other quantitative and even qualitative designs can be synthesised. For example, and more recently, these methods have been utilised to synthesise qualitative research evidence (Thomas and Harden, 2008). This type of synthesis, pooled or filtered study is referred to as a systematic review and/or meta-analysis, depending upon the level of re-analysis of the data from the included studies.

A systematic review should not be confused with a literature review, as it is a research design in its own right, which involves the systematic searching of the published and unpublished literature on the topic of interest and combining the results, when appropriate, to give a more precise picture of the effectiveness of a treatment, intervention or programme than can be provided by an individual study (Centre for Reviews and Dissemination, 2009). While a systematic review also involves the systematic gathering and reviewing of research evidence on a particular topic, it also requires stringent adherence to the research protocol, which details specific procedures utilised to retrieve and analyse the information. Strict adherence is crucial, as the review must be reproducible. In short, review methodologies are positioned at the top of the hierarchy for their ability to pool evidence from single studies, essentially increasing the sample size in order to provide a more reliable estimate of effectiveness.

Level I–2: Randomised controlled trial

The RCT is considered to be the 'gold standard' in clinical and biomedical research for its ability to eradicate and control for biases that might impact on the research outcomes. An RCT design is used to assess the effectiveness of treatments and interventions (Carr *et al.*, 2007; Centre for Reviews and Dissemination, 2009). As indicated above, there are several key characteristics that distinguish an RCT from other experimental and non-experimental designs. These include the presence of two or more treatment or intervention groups, one of which does not receive the treatment or intervention, also known as the control group, and the random allocation of participants to control and intervention groups, meaning that all participants in the study have an equal chance of being allocated to one of the groups. Another distinguishing feature of the RCT design is the comparison of the groups based on achievement or performance in relation to outcome measure (Carr *et al.*, 2007).

The use of such a research design is, when feasible, the most appropriate for assessing whether or not the treatment or intervention tested is better suited for producing the desired outcome rather than those receiving no treatment or intervention. Because of the random allocation of participants to control and intervention groups, the likelihood that the observed outcomes are a result of the intervention can be more reliably assessed and it is less likely that the observed results occurred due to chance or bias associated with the allocation of participants.

RCTs also use large sample sizes, allowing the intervention to be tested on a large number of people; the larger the numbers, the less likely the observed results are achieved by chance.

In addition to the traditional RCT design, there are other variations, such as multicentred trails, where the same trial is carried out at multiple sites or 'centres', and community trials, which are a type of cluster randomised trials. Community or cluster randomised trials are often utilised when random allocation of individuals is not possible or when concerned with population level indicators. Clusters or groups are randomly allocated to the intervention or control groups. Cluster randomisation is also advised when access to the sampling frame or the list of all eligible participants is not available in order to ensure that the observed outcomes are not affected or biased by participant allocation.

Non-randomised controlled trial designs, such as before-and-after studies and interrupted time series studies, can also be utilised to assess the effectiveness of a proposed intervention; however due to the lack of randomisation of participation, this increases the risk of bias (Centre for Reviews and Dissemination, 2009).

The next level of evidence, Level II, is occupied by several designs commonly utilised in public health research. As these designs do not employ a random allocation of participants or populations to groups, and do not seek to intervene, but rather observe and measure a phenomenon, they occupy positions below that of the RCT on the hierarchy. Rather than force or allocate comparison groups, these studies measure a natural or observed difference between the groups of interest. Studies employing this type of design are referred to as observational studies. In various ways they examine the effect of an intervention or exposure to an intervention on a health outcome and provide some measure of this relationship or association (Carr *et al.*, 2007). These various designs are explored in further detail below.

Level II-1: Cohort design

The first of the observational designs occupying the second tier of the hierarchy is the cohort design. A cohort study involves following a set population group over time, and similar to the designs discussed above, a comparison is made between groups that received and those that did not receive the intervention to ascertain whether or not exposure is related to the intervention. This group or groups are followed over time, often in public health research to compare the incidence of the health outcome in each group (Carr *et al.*, 2007). A cohort study brings to light the association between exposure and outcome, but cannot establish a causal relationship. For example, as Pisani (2008) explained when trying to debunk the myth that needle exchange programmes caused HIV infections in the 1990s in Vancouver, the answer could only be provided by following a cohort of non-HIV-infected injecting drug users to see if exposure to needle exchange programmes led to an HIV infection.

Unlike an RCT, a cohort study makes some steps towards providing an explanation for intervention or health outcomes, but establishing whether or not an association is 'real', rather than artefact requires further investigation.

Level II-2: Case-control design

Similar to the cohort study, in its ability to provide further evidence of causal relationships, a case–control study utilises comparison groups, but the aim is to evaluate the association between exposure to an intervention and the outcome. Case–control studies in public health often compare people with a particular characteristic of interest (e.g. a particular disease) with those people without it. Those with the disease are referred to as the 'case', while those without the disease are referred to as the 'control'. For example, Fajo-Pascual *et al.* (2010) used a case–control study to explore the risk factors for *Campylobacter* infections (a type of food poisoning). They found that risk factors such as eating chicken three or more times a week or eating meat from a deli counter with poor hygiene control were strongly associated with poisoning.

The strength of the association between the outcome and risk of the outcome (exposure) is measured by calculating the odds ratio. Calculating the odds ratio tells you about the risk of an outcome based on exposure, but does not tell you about the incidence of disease in the exposed population. Without taking into account the 'incident cases' (new) and excluding 'prevalent cases' (existing) and selecting the case and control groups independent of exposure status, a case–control study will be unable to provide a valid estimate of relative risk (Carr *et al.*, 2007). It is for this reason and that case–control studies are also prone to other types of bias, such as information bias, particularly recall bias, which positions case–control studies further down the hierarchy.

Level II–3: Cross-sectional design

Cross-sectional studies, which in public health are classed as either ecological or descriptive studies depending on how the gathered information is analysed, are usually conducted using routinely collected data to explore the associations between diseases and possible causes. These study designs are also used to establish disease prevalence (in prevalence surveys). This type of study provides a snapshot at one time point, and is unable distinguish the direction of the relationship between the disease and its cause (i.e. does obesity cause diabetes or does diabetes cause obesity?), but are seen as a good way to generate ideas about possible causation. Because of the inability to establish a certain link between disease/health condition to one or more causal factors, results from cross-sectional studies are said to be inconclusive and act as a starting point for further inquiry.

Level II–4: Case series design

Case series designs differ from the other study designs described above in that there is no comparison group. Rather this design provides a description of a number of cases in which an intervention was implemented or a condition was observed along with the reported outcomes. These types of studies are also referred to as 'case reports' as they tend to describe cases which stand out from the usual picture. By design, these studies are used to test new hypotheses or to study new/emerging diseases and because of the lack of a control group and the inability to assess the frequency of exposure to risk factor, the design is seen to be more prone to bias. This explains its position as the lowest of all experimental research designs in the Level II hierarchy.

Level III: Well-designed non-experimental studies

This level is occupied by evidence from studies that do not involve hypothesis testing or experimentation. It is unclear whether or not qualitative research falls into this category or if it is still reserved for descriptive quantitative research. Descriptive studies which normally answer questions about 'the frequency of health states and their known and possible causes by person, place and time' (Carr et al., 2007, page 58). Descriptive studies are able to provide evidence about the age of a particular population experiencing a particular health state, the geography of particular health states and the frequency or change in health states over time. In addition, many descriptive studies utilise routinely collected data, which means that the data do not need to be collected in every case. Other types of studies that fit into this category include surveys and qualitative research.

In terms of qualitative research evidence, some propose that a separate hierarchy is needed in order to differentiate between the various methodological approaches and designs. This hierarchy is structured around the ability of different types and designs of studies to produce 'transferable evidence, evidence that is generalizable beyond the setting of where the study is conducted' (Daly *et al.*, 2007, page 45). Thus, studies at the top of this qualitative hierarchy are studies which are generalisable, followed by conceptual studies, descriptive studies and then single-case studies.

Levels IV and V

Towards the end of the hierarchy, Levels IV and V, there is a noticeable absence of empirical research and research evidence. Level IV acknowledges that in every case there may not be the available research evidence or the opportunity to collect this evidence by recognising the use and importance of professional or expert opinion. While professional expertise does carry weight, it cannot form the basis for changing practice or initiating an intervention. Without empirical evidence to support such knowledge, the information is largely experiential and potentially laden with biases.

The final rung on the evidential ladder, and by some accounts the anti-thesis to evidence-based practice, is the equivalent to scientific hearsay or gossip, in essence based on no sound or empirical evidence. While what you may have heard or been told might be interesting or likely to be accurate, without research evidence to provide support, the 'someone told me' is unlikely to be used to inform or change practice.

Now that you have a better idea of the various types of study designs that occupy the evidential hierarchy, you may wonder how the positions of the various types of evidence on the hierarchy impact on the evidence's ability to inform or change practice, the point of evidence-based practice and evidence-based public health. Watterson and Watterson (2003) argue that a researcher's position in relation to the hierarchy and credence given to evidence that is lower ranked or absent is largely informed by the research tradition within one's discipline. Thus, the usefulness of the currently accepted hierarchy and its assumptions about what constitutes evidence and knowledge pay homage to the clinical and medical influences within public health and the relevance of clinical or biomedical evidence to informing one's practice. Its use in a multi-disciplinary field such as public health often requires the consideration of many different levels of evidence.

Case study 3.1: The birth of the Cochrane Collaboration

As research and clinical practice developed, vast amounts of information became available to health care practitioners; the sheer volume of this made it difficult to access and assimilate this information/evidence effectively and find the best evidence in order to make well-informed health care decisions.

In response to this information overload and the need to access and assimilate the most effective and efficient evidence, Archie Cochrane developed the Cochrane database in the early 1970s. The database collated data from RCTs, deemed the best evidence for indicating effectiveness, in order to streamline researcher and practitioner access to information. This system led to the development of the systematic review methodology of pooling together RCT evidence for decision making, which is now recognised as the highest level of available research evidence.

The Cochrane database also evolved to provide health care practitioners with a store or register of research on the efficacy of various care options and also a critical insight into evidence provided by RCTs indicating whether the various studies were effective, ineffective or of unknown value.

With the arrival of the internet the Cochrane database led to the development of the online Cochrane Library, a widely used resource for health care practitioners, policy makers and patients. The Library is a part of the Cochrane Collaboration, an international non-profit organisation set up in 1993 and dedicated to making well-informed decisions about human health care.

Visit the Cochrane Collaboration to learn more about its history and the resources available in the Library: www.cochrane.org.

Using the hierarchy

When looking for evidence to help inform decision making, we should look for the highest level of evidence available, but also the best-quality evidence, to answer the research question of interest (Gillam *et al.*, 2007). As discussed previously, certain research designs are better suited for addressing certain types of research questions. This means that not every research question can be answered with an RCT, nor can every research question be answered quantitatively. An RCT can answer research questions about the effectiveness of an intervention, and no other study design is able to answer this type of research question, for example a cohort design does not encompass and intervention component, therefore, is an inappropriate design to use if you want to know whether or not a healthy eating intervention in primary schools has been effective in getting students to eat more fruit and vegetables. You simply would not be able answer your research question in utilising this type of design; however, utilising cohort design you would be able to explore the association between exposure to healthy eating programmes or interventions that had an impact on the food choices of school children.

Similarly, if you want to answer a research question that is concerned with finding out the cause of a disease, case–control or cohort studies provide the best and only options for answering this type of research question. Thus, navigating your way through the evidence-based practice field is less about looking for or designing an RCT to address your research question, but more about finding and/or using the most appropriate and most reliable evidence, whatever the level.

ACTIVITY 3.2

Read the scenario below and reflect on the options provided and reflect on how or if the hierarchy of evidence influenced your decision.

You are an epidemiologist working for the Health Protection Agency and you are asked to provide evidence for or against rolling out a new vaccine for Hepatitis B in a high-risk population group. You know that several empirical studies have been conducted to examine the effectiveness of this new Hepatitis B vaccine in several populations, including those considered to be at the highest risk for infection, but you are not sure how effective this new vaccination is a preventing contraction of Hepatitis B with potential exposure and if you should be advocating for utilising the new vaccination, which is more expensive than the old one. You also need to know whether or not this new vaccination, which requires a series of follow-ups, will be acceptable among all of the high-risk groups, particularly transitory populations.

What do you do?

- *Option A*: Guess. After all, you have lots of expertise in the area, and both you and your colleagues have an idea about which vaccination you think is most effective. So, what harm can an educated guess be?
- *Option B*: Conduct a structured and thorough search of the empirical research and pool together findings from relevant interventions in order to compare the effect of the old and new vaccines in terms of desired outcome and cost-effectiveness. You base your decision on the evidence gathered without first appraising – after all, the evidence is published and peer reviewed – and pool together the evidence from several RCTs.
- *Option C*: Re-examine the data gathered not just in terms of the intervention effects or the significance reported in terms of outcome measures. Each survey must be assessed for methodological quality, as well as the reliability of the outcome reported.

Comment: There are many sources of information that you could draw upon to help make your decision; you need to draw upon published research evidence. Consult the evidential hierarchy to help decide what type of research evidence to use; however, if time and resources are limited, conducting a randomised control trial or a systematic review is not feasible. Perhaps there is already a published systematic review or RCTs examining this topic which would be helpful for making a decision.

Limitations of the hierarchy towards assessing methodological quality and rigour

We now have a better idea of the various research designs and the level of evidence provided. We have also seen how you might utilise the hierarchy to guide your decision making. Next, we will briefly explore the limitations and the need to go further in order to assess the quality of evidence, rather than relying on the type of design to tell us about the quality of the research. The limitations of the hierarchy largely centre on assumptions about methodological quality and rigour. While the hierarchy argues that research design provides strength and reliability of evidence, a study's design alone is not sufficient to judge its quality. The use of study design alone cannot determine or predict the credibility of the evidence and many critics argue that the current system fails to address both a study's reliability and credibility in terms of concept and delivery (Rychetnik *et al.*, 2002; Petticrew and Roberts, 2003). While an intervention may tick all the appropriate methodological boxes to put it at the top of the list in theory, the study's ability to deliver reliable outcomes is equally important.

Baum (2010) argues that public health research should be focused less on attaining methodological purity and more on utilising the most appropriate research approaches, no matter how eclectic, to answer research questions that shape policy and practice. With any type of research it is not only the methodology chosen, but also adherence to methodological principles that impact on its rigour and reliability. Just because a study has employed an RCT design, which is said to provide the second most reliable source of evidence, it does not mean that it will automatically be a well-executed piece of research. Similarly, it should not be assumed that all studies employing the same research design are equal in weighting or that they are well conducted. Poorly conducted research is just as ineffective for decision-making purposes as no evidence at all, and it is imprudent and often costly to base decision making on limited or poor evidence.

Moving beyond the label and association of research design requires assessing the actual quality of the research. Assessing quality involves issues of validity (internal and external) as well as the reliability of the outcomes presented. The act of assessing the validity and reliability of research is called 'critical appraisal' and has become a vital skill or step in evidence-based medicine and public health decision making. The steps and skills important for critical appraisal will be discussed in detail in the next chapter.

ACTIVITY 3.3 REVISING OR DEVISING A NEW HIERARCHY

Take a few moments to think about how you might like to revise the hierarchy of evidence to take into account the study's design and quality. Or perhaps you would like to devise a new hierarchy.

- What criteria would you add or change in the existing hierarchy?
- What would an entirely new hierarchy look like?

Chapter summary

The hierarchy of evidence is used to rank methodological approaches or study designs based on their propensity towards and handling of methodological bias or reliability which is likely to impact on the observed outcomes or findings of the research. Within this framework, study designs are assigned to levels. In the hierarchy presented in this chapter there were five levels of evidence arranged from the most reliable (systematic reviews) to the least reliable (someone told me ...). Planning useful, practice-focused public health research requires drawing on existing research evidence while utilising a wider theoretical lens for viewing and appreciating public health evidence. Ultimately, the most useful and most reliable research evidence is evidence that can lend the best solutions to practice-based problems, and the judging of the quality of this evidence should be guided by, but not solely by, the evidential hierarchy.

GOING FURTHER

In order to further extend your knowledge of the information presented in this chapter, you may want to look for more examples of the various study designs described above. You may also want to further engage with the debate around the use and utility of the hierarchy of evidence. Some useful for resources for exploring this debate include:

- Blum, R (2009) Some observations on 'observational' research. *Perspectives in Biology and Medicine*, 52(2): 252–263.

- Concato, J, Shah, N and Horwitz, R (2000) Randomized, Controlled Trials, Observational Studies and the Hierarchy of Research Designs. *New England Journal of Medicine*, 342(25): 1887–1892.

- Ho, PM, Peterson, P and Masoudi, F (2008) Evaluating the evidence: is there a rigid hierarchy? *Circulation*, 118: 1675–1684.

- Merlin, T, Weston, A and Tooher, R (2009) Extending the hierarchy to include topics other than treatment: revising the Australian 'levels of evidence. *BMC Medical Research Methodology*, 9: 34.

chapter 4

The Act/Art of Assessing: Critical Appraisal and its Relevance in Public Health
Nena Foster

Meeting the public health competences

Core area 2: Assessing the evidence of effectiveness of interventions, programmes and services to improve population health and wellbeing

This chapter will help you to evidence the following competences for public health (Public Health Skills and Careers Framework):

- Level 6 (b) Knowledge of the principles of critical appraisal as applied to various studies and its use in improving health and wellbeing
- Level 7 (a) Understanding of appraising the quality of primary and secondary research.

This chapter will also assist you in demonstrating the following National Occupational Standard(s) for public health:

- Assess the evidence and impact of health and health care – (PHS07) interventions, programmes and services and apply the assessments to practice
- Improve the quality of health and health care interventions and services through audit and evaluation – (PHS08)
- Support and challenge workers on specific aspects of their practice – (CJ F309).

This chapter will also be useful in demonstrating Standards 4c and 4e and 7 of the Public Health Practitioner Standards:

- Standard 4. Continually develop and improve own and others' practice in public health by:

  d. the application of evidence in improving own area of work
  e. objectively and constructively contributing to reviewing the effectiveness of own area of work.

- Standard 7. Assess the evidence of effective interventions and services to improve health and wellbeing – demonstrating:

  a. knowledge of the different types, sources and levels of evidence in own area of practice and how to access and use them
  b. the appraisal of published evidence and the identification of implications for own area of work practice.

Chapter overview

This chapter builds on the knowledge from the previous chapter about the various types and strength of evidence, and builds on the notion of judging research evidence based on the research design, as well as the adherence to and utilisation of the prescribed methodological principles. This chapter will define the process of judging the quality of research, explain the significance of this activity for public health research and practice, and discuss the processes, tools and resources available for these purposes.

Exercises in this chapter will focus on:

- developing an understanding of what is meant by critical appraisal;
- building skills for conducting a critical appraisal;
- developing skills in choosing appropriate tools for critical appraisal.

Learning outcomes

After reading this chapter you will be able to:

- explain what is meant by critical appraisal;
- select appropriate tools for and carry out a critical appraisal;
- locate appropriate information from public health research studies, and assess the quality of the information presented.

What is critical appraisal?

Chapter 1 provided a brief introduction to this concept, which this chapter will explore in more detail. As a postgraduate student and/or a health professional you will be familiar with the latest and breaking research in your specialist area; however, you may or may not have had the opportunity to engage with this information and you may think, 'what does all of this mean?' or 'how does this affect my practice?' Critical appraisal literally describes the process and skills needed to judge or 'appraise' the quality of research evidence and the process of scrutinising or 'critical' investigation of this evidence. As Burls (2009, page 1) describes it, critical appraisal is careful and systematic as a process, and is focused on judging the 'trustworthiness' and relevance of research evidence to practice. This means that these are key skills for those working in public health as well as other contexts where decision making must be based on reliable and relevant evidence.

Critical appraisal aims to assess the shortcomings of research evidence, mostly evidence that has been published in peer-reviewed academic texts and journals. However, not all research is conducted rigorously, and while all research has its limitations or shortcomings, it is important that these are identified and it is the job of the appraiser to decide whether or not these limitations, such as biases, impact on the quality and utility of the research findings. In essence, is the research flawed, but still providing usable information? It is also the job of the assessor or appraiser to decide the impact of these limitations on the research findings and whether or not these limitations could have been avoided or mitigated. Essentially, critical appraisal seeks to establish whether or not a researcher has done all that is possible to produce the most reliable results, given the research design and 'real world' circumstances, in order to mitigate or minimise instances of bias. It is also the job of the appraiser to assess whether or not these biases impact on the results observed. Crombie (1996, page 2) argues that all research has flaws and something can be learned from all studies, even if it is how not to utilise a particular research design. Thus, there is no 'bad' research, but rather better or worse research for informing practice and decision making.

The purpose and significance of critical appraisal in public health

The purpose of critical appraisal in public health may seem obvious, but might also seem unnecessary given that much of the evidence has been published. As practitioners are involved in decision making, increasingly at the policy-making level, it is important to be able to read and scrutinise research in everyday practice but also to argue for public health policy change is crucial. It would be difficult to argue for practice or policy change without reliable evidence to support your ideas.

Again, it might seem clear why critical appraisal is necessary, but still unclear as to why or how you can argue with published research results. Despite the peer-review process for health research, a process which involves review of the research by other expert researchers in the field or trained journal staff, publication is not synonymous with rigour and practicability or relevance. While this process of peer review may be better at weeding out the less rigorous research, it perhaps is less useful for deciding what is most relevant in a practice setting. As critical appraisal is concerned with both rigour and relevance, the usefulness of research for improving practice is equally important. It is important for public health professionals to have the skills necessary to decide whether or not research evidence is rigorous, relevant and can be used to improve health status and health outcomes. In addition, public health professionals must understand and have the skills necessary to maximise health outcomes, but also to avoid making untrue and potentially misleading claims – a potentially dangerous situation depending on the stake.

ACTIVITY 4.1

Reflect on the 'if you can't prove it's not true, then it's not untrue' philosophy often employed in the sale of consumer goods to answer the following questions:

- Why might this be a problematic approach for public health practitioners?
- How might an advocate for critical appraisal poke holes in this claim?

Comment: Public health interventions need to be based on evidence of effectiveness and where this is not available they should be based on best practice. Unlike the sale of consumer goods, a public health intervention can have important consequences for population health and wellbeing. Employing an 'if you can't prove it's not true, then it's not untrue' approach to public health would be ethically wrong and potentially harmful. An advocate for critical appraisal would argue that evidence of what works and what doesn't is needed and should be used to underpin any public health programme.

Getting started: building the necessary skills for conducting critical appraisal

By now you will have some insight into what critical appraisal entails and what skills are needed. You should also have a better understanding of the various research designs from the previous chapter, and be able to distinguish one research design from another. And soon, you will have the confidence to interrogate published research, once the skills needed and the process is explained. A good working knowledge of the various research methodologies and designs is crucial to precritical appraisal learning. It is important to understand the various principles associated with the methodology designs and their limitations in order to judge whether or not the research has rigorously upheld these principles and perhaps how the researchers could have done things more rigorously.

The first step in appraising research is, of course, finding the relevant research. For the purpose of this chapter we will assume you already know how to do this. Then you need to be able to read and make sense of what you read, before being able to appraise it. Greenhalgh's (2004) 'How to read a paper' is a useful starter text for helping to familiarise yourself with the commonly used presentation formats of scientific research and for finding your way around various types of research articles. Knowing how research is formatted will help you to find the signposts for the necessary information. According to Greenhalgh (2004) the IMRAD (Introduction, Methods, Results and Discussion) format is most commonly used in the presentation of scientific information, making it much easier to locate the information required to perform the appraisal. All of these sections and the corresponding information should be present in the article that you are appraising. Missing, misplaced or incomplete information make the task more difficult. In particular, if a study's methods are unclear or unreported, then deciding the appropriate criteria for appraising research will pose a problem. Poor description or unreported research methods is a common flaw, and it often deals a fatal blow to the study's quality. In addition, remembering the mnemonic PICO (Patient, Intervention, Comparator, and Outcome) as suggested by Makela and Witt (2005), will help you find your way around particular types of studies with interventional designs. Being able to understand and locate these various components of the intervention will aid in appraising.

It is not only important to locate the appropriate information, but you must also assess the quality of the information presented. In order to do this you must ask several evaluative questions, and these evaluative questions usually require you to appraise several aspects of the research such as:

- Rationale and purpose of the study (e.g. Is the purpose stated? Does this study seem appropriate?)

- Study design (e.g. Is this study designed to collect the appropriate data to answer the designated research question(s)?)

- Analysis of the data (e.g. Are the significant variables actually significant? Has the data been analysed according to the stated methodological conventions?)

- Study discussion/conclusions (e.g. Do the conclusions match the research undertaken?).

(Oliver and Peersman, 2001, pages 85–86)

While most research papers are published in the IMRAD or a similar format, it is important to note that not all research will be presented neatly. Finding the information that you need to conduct your appraisal may require some picking through, hunting and wading in, but a good appraiser first finds the all of the evidence before making a judgement about the research's quality. Being able to read and understand what you read is perhaps the most important skill required for critical appraisal, and as mentioned above requires good working knowledge of various research methodologies.

The second most important skill is remaining objective or neutral while appraising your research. As human beings we all have individual preferences about how we prefer information to be presented; however, critical appraisal is not about 'trashing' or slating the work of others. It is important to recognise that all studies fall short of the 'golden ideal' and should be appraised in the light of what they have been able to achieve. Remaining objective is about thinking realistically. Most studies will have deficiencies but, given the particular circumstances, could the research have been improved? The evidence they provide may not always be strong but, if it is the best that is likely to be available, we should not immediately discount it because of the flaws. It is perhaps more useful to draw from it what information we can. So, be cautious, even-handed and logical in your assessment of published research and remember, critical appraisal serves as a reminder that just because a study has been published it does not mean that its findings should be accepted blindly.

In order to begin assessing the quality of the evidence presented in one or more studies you will first need to familiarise yourself with the information presented. The study's abstract may be your first port of call, but it may not always provide the detail needed, meaning you have to read further into the text. Girden (1996) discusses the various aspects of a study to be examined when evaluating research, such as the study's purpose or rationale, the design, analysis of the data and author's conclusions. Conducting a thorough reading of the research paper is the only way to locate this information.

As your task is not only to locate these various bit of information, but also to judge how well the information is presented and how rigorously the study was undertaken, your work does not stop there. Perhaps the next the step and yet another skill necessary for conducting critical appraisal is locating and examining the study's research design, often found in the 'Methods' section. This section of the paper often holds the secret to what types of questions you will need to ask of the research in order to provide a critical, yet fair appraisal. In order to know what types of questions should be asked of the research, the methods, while a subject of scrutiny, also dictate the type of critical appraisal aide or tool that should be used to interrogate the research.

ACTIVITY 4.2

Take a few moments to think about and list the skills necessary for conducting critical appraisal. Indicate why you think these skills are important.

Comment: You might have considered the importance of remaining neutral and the ability to think in a systematic way. Alternatively, you might have considered the need to ask searching and appropriate questions of the research. All of these skills are essential as is the ability to consider the relevance of the research and the applicability of the study findings.

Assessing research quality and relevance

Critical appraisal is not just about assessing the research quality, but is also concerned with the significance or relevance of the findings and whether or not the study's findings can inform or change practice. In terms of quantitative research, determining quality is associated with the notions of reliability and validity. Essentially, based on how the research has been described to be carried out, is it likely that the observed results are not produced by chance. This requires close examination of several components of the study's design, such as:

- Sample size (Was there any bias in the sample selection? Is the sample size large enough to produce statistically significant results?)

- Outcome measures (Are these clearly defined and measured appropriately? Were all relevant outcome measures included? Was there any misclassification of outcome measures and how might this have impacted on the study's results?)

- Statistical analysis (Was this clearly reported? Are the confidence intervals reported? What is the probability that the results have occurred by chance rather than there being a real effect?)

- Confounders (Were these accounted or controlled for? How might these have impacted on the study's results?).

Once the parameters above have been judged, you will be able to assess the internal and external validity of the research – the ultimate test of the quality of the research. A study is considered to be internally valid if it has achieved what it has set out to achieve, accounted for its limitations and its conclusions are justified and within the scope of the research. External validity is equally important as all quantitative study designs should generate research results that are generalisable wider than the study population to the target population. Only if a study has achieved internal validity can it be considered externally valid. In short, the appraiser must be convinced that the study, as it was carried out and reported, produced results that are reliable and applicable to other similar populations.

Judging the significance or relevance of research involves more than looking for statistically significant findings. In terms of quantitative research, while p-values can provide evidence for or against the null-hypothesis, they often tell us very little about size or direction of the effect observed. It may also be the case that statistical significance does not translate into clinical significance, meaning variables that exhibit a statistical significance may be impossible or too small to warrant practice or policy change. Conversely, there can be clinical significance without statistical significance, which can occur if the sample size utilised is too small to generate statistically significant results. In short, significance is not about simply finding statistical significance, which can lead to clinical significance, but the two are not necessarily mutually exclusive. And, as clinical significance is important, the findings must be relevant to the context in which they are to be applied if practice or policy change is to be initiated, we should not base decisions about significance solely on statistical significance.

Similarly, in qualitative research you must assess the study's design along similar parameters, taking into account the chosen research methodology, the data collection methods, the interpretation of the results and the conclusions reached. In terms of qualitative research judging significance of a study is about whether or not the study's findings are worth taking note of or paying attention to, for example, does the research present findings which are novel, interesting and relevant to the context of interest. Rather than being solely concerned with issues of reliability and validity, qualitative research is judged by the notion of 'trustworthiness'. Lincoln and Guba (1985) categorise 'trustworthiness' by four parameters:

- Credibility (Are the research findings a likely or 'credible' interpretation of the data, i.e. is it the interpretation plausible?)

- Transferability (Can the findings from the study transfer beyond this study?)

- Dependability (Is there a harmony between the data collection tools, data analysis, the theory generated and the theoretical perspective?)

- Conformability (Are the study's findings supported by the data collected?).

Finding the right critical appraisal tool

By now it should come as no surprise to you to learn that the designs of quantitative and qualitative studies differ, and that you will need to differentiate between quantitative and qualitative research designs. Because of these design differences, there are specific evaluative questions you will need to ask to appraise these different types of research (Crombie, 1996). Whether or not you come up with your own tool based on a set of evaluative questions appropriate for the study's design or make use of an already developed tool, you must ask the appropriate evaluative questions. For example, using an appraisal tool or set appraisal questions designed to appraise a quantitative study is not appropriate for evaluating a qualitative study. Similarly, using an evaluative tool for a randomised controlled trial (RCT) is not appropriate for evaluating a cohort study, both of which are quantitative study designs but employ different quantitative methodological principles (see Chapter 3 for a fuller explanation of these principles).

If you want to make use of existing critical appraisal tools, there are several which have been developed. In this chapter we will focus on those specifically developed for public health research.

A number of critical appraisal skills programmes have been developed, together with a set of useful and easy-to-use tools that provide evaluative questions for the appraisal of different types of research studies relevant for public health research. These tools are widely used and readily available on the internet and include tools for appraising a range of study designs (i.e. systematic reviews, RCTs, economic evaluations, cohort studies, case–control studies, diagnostic studies and qualitative research studies).

For example, the former Public Health Resource Unit's Critical Appraisal Skills Programme tools use 10–12 questions to guide you through your appraisal. These questions are often 'tick box' style questions, which require you as the appraiser to justify your answer.

In addition, Heller *et al.* (2008) have developed a checklist for public health research. This checklist, much like the CASP tools, guides the appraiser through a set of steps designed to appraise the quality of a study, including examining the research question and the study's design/data collection methods. This tool can be simplified into four steps: 'ask', 'collect', 'understand' and 'use', and sets itself apart from other critical appraisal tools in being more relevant for public health research as it seeks to 'understand' the population relevance of the results as well 'use' or apply these results in a public health setting. The authors of this framework argue that it is specifically designed and useful for public health interventions, rather than clinical interventions, and can also be used to appraise studies addressing public health policy issues.

ACTIVITY 4.3

After reading the abstract below, think about the most appropriate appraisal questions to ask in appraising this research.

Background: Although several plausible biological mechanisms have been advanced for the association between greater physical stature and lower

---

coronary heart disease (CHD) risk in prospective cohort studies, the importance of one of the principal artefactual explanations – reverse causality due to shrinkage – remains unresolved. To explore this issue, studies with repeat measurements of height are required, but, to date, such data have been lacking. **Objective**: To examine the possible relationship between height loss and future CHD. Methods: Data were analysed from the Whitehall II study of 3802 men and 1615 women who participated in a physical examination in 1985–8, had their height re-measured in 1997–9, and were then followed up for fatal and non-fatal CHD. **Results**: A mean follow-up of 7.4 years after the second height measurement gave rise to 69 CHD events in men and 18 in women. After adjustment for baseline CHD risk factors, greater loss of physical stature between survey and resurvey was associated with an increased risk of CHD in men (HR; 95 per cent CI for a one SD increase: 1.24; 1.00 to 1.53) but not women (0.93; 0.58 to 1.50). **Conclusions**: Reverse causality due to shrinkage may contribute to the inverse association between a single measurement of height and later CHD in other studies.

(Adapted from Batty *et al.* (2010) Height loss and future coronary heart disease in London: the Whitehall II study. *Journal of Epidemiology and Community Health*, Aug 30.)

Comment: In the abstract this study is identified as using a cohort study design. In addition to asking some appraisal questions specifically about this type of research design, you might also ask some more general questions about the research. Some appropriate appraisal questions might include:

- Did the study have a clear focus?
- Was the chosen research design appropriate for answering the research question?
- Was the cohort recruited in an acceptable way (e.g. was the representative of a defined population or was everyone included that should have been included)?
- Was the exposure accurately measured in order to minimise bias?
- Was the outcome measured in order to minimise bias?

Also useful is the compilation of critical appraisal tools for public health practice by Ciliska *et al.* (2008). This report provides information on and links to some of the more commonly used guidelines and checklists used by public health professionals.

Applying the appraisal tool and crafting robust critiques

Deciding whether or not the results or findings from a study are useful for informing or changing practice can involve using a checklist or critical appraisal tool, but using a checklist is not a substitution for thinking through and justifying your critiques of the appraised study. These simply provide a guideline to help you get started and become accustomed to the types of information and questions that you need to ask of the study in order to appraise it. If you are using a checklist or tool to help, you must still reach a final verdict about the soundness of the research after having reviewed various components of the study as guided by the tool or checklist.

The act of appraisal becomes a bit of an art as you judge various elements of the study individually, while simultaneously judging the whole and in order to craft critiques of the research which justify your verdict. If you conclude that a study does not provide sound or good evidence, you must be able to indicate how and why you came to this verdict, this is conversely true if you decide that the level of evidence is sound and useful for informing practice. It is not sufficient to say that the study provides 'good evidence' and not say why it provides good evidence; this would be contrary to the practice of evidence-based public health. You must not only deliver a final verdict, but you must also justify your conclusions and support your decisions.

In order to support your decision and justify the critiques that you have formulated you must make use of and draw on other relevant research, clinical or methodological evidence for support. It is also important, as we said earlier in the chapter, to be objective, and it is equally important, particularly in crafting critiques of the research, to be critical but fair. You might ask, how can I be critical without pulling apart or being seen to be damning the work of other researchers? This involves being cautious, which means refraining from jumping to any conclusions about the quality of the research prematurely. Foregone conclusions are especially important to avoid. For example, you must read beyond the abstract of a paper to fully and cautiously assess the study's quality. Likewise, you should not undertake an appraisal with your mind already made up about the study's quality. This may sound obvious, but it is important to be aware of potential biases that the appraiser might experience. For example, the 'halo effect' – where a study conducted by well-known researchers might be viewed more favourably than research from less or unknown researchers – would impact on the appraiser's ability to remain objective. As mentioned previously, published research does not equate to rigorous research, even if it comes from an imminent or experienced research team. In addition to being cautious, it is also important to be even-handed in your critiques of the study. There will be some limitations, but it is important to note what can be learned from the study despite its limitations; there is always something.

Finally, it is important to be logical and realistic in your assessment of what the study could or should have achieved and how it could be improved. For example, it would be unrealistic to suggest that the researchers should undertake an RCT, when this is neither a feasible or appropriate design for answering the research query. This critique is not only impractical, it also demonstrates a poor understanding of research design.

Now that you perhaps have a better understanding of what it means to be 'critical' you might require some help coming up with suitable or appropriate critiques. The list below provides some suggestions to help you create a well-structured and well-supported appraisal.

- Structure the whole appraisal and your critiques even-handedly.

  – Highlight the good and the bad: What worked well/did not work well? Why?

  – Use the areas for appraisal to provide structure for your written appraisal.

- Justify your critiques.

  – Critique: X is problematic. Why is X problematic? How could it be improved upon?

- Use evidence from the study as well as other studies to provide support.

  – Give page numbers; quote the study directly.

  – Utilise other relevant research.

Again, the tips presented above are merely to help guide you in formulating your appraisal and critiques. You are still required to do the thinking and writing. Have a look at the next activity, to help illustrate how an appropriate critique might look.

ACTIVITY 4.4

Read the following three example critiques and decide which of these is an appropriate (or a more appropriate) critique? Explain why.

- The study's methods are interesting and good.
- The researchers should not have bothered with this research; its findings are insignificant.
- The sample was deemed sufficient to collect 'sufficiently rich data'; however, the data collection methods generated a largely homogenous sample.

  Comment: Of the three critiques above there may appear to be an obviously correct answer. Not only is the final critique objective, balanced and fair, it takes into account several of the key aspects of research that you must examine when undertaking an appraisal (i.e. the study sample, methods and the analysis of the data).

Common flaws encountered when appraising

Fortunately, or perhaps unfortunately, researchers can be rather predictable in the mistakes made while researching and are similarly constrained by the same 'real world' issues that impact on the research environment. Research involving human participation is less predictable than research undertaken in the controlled environment of a laboratory, but nevertheless, good researchers are able to control for or minimise the impact of these flaws on the research and at the very least these are declared or stated in the study's reporting. A study's limitations are usually stated in the 'Discussion' or 'Conclusion' section; however, it is important to note that there are potentially unstated limitations, and it is just as important to identify the flaws or limitations as it is to assess the impact or the magnitude of this impact on the study's findings and overall quality.

Some of the common flaws, which may or may not be declared by the researchers, include: mismeasured, misreported or missing key findings; bias; chance; confounders; lack of rigour. These are explained below. With practice, it will become easier to spot these flaws and convey their potential impact on the quality of evidence provided by the study.

The first common flaw identified above – misreported or missing key findings – is perhaps less likely than the others to be identified by the researcher(s) as one of the study's limitations as it is either unintentional or unknown to the researcher or could potentially mask a larger problem, perhaps with the research design. This flaw can occur for several reasons. It could be that the research does not investigate or measure what it sets out in its research question, aims or objectives. This may result in reporting key findings which do not follow from the research. Sometimes human error in calculation or data entry can lead to statistical errors and these errors are then reported as findings. In qualitative research, poor or unverified coding systems may lead to misinterpretation of data and subsequently the findings are flawed.

The second flaw identified above is that of bias. As we have discussed, bias comes in many forms, whether it is bias in selecting the sample or in the measurement of the phenomenon of interest. Quantitative researchers should seek to eliminate bias and qualitative researchers should acknowledge the bias. In many cases, bias is avoidable, but when it is not, or in the case of qualitative research part of the research's uniqueness, it must be declared.

While bias is often imposed by the researcher, chance is not, as it results from random variation. Assuring that the observed results of the study are not due to chance or luck for quantitative research is crucial, as a study with results largely achieved by random does not make good or generalisable evidence. Some mechanisms noted in the previous chapter in the discussion of study designs that help to minimise or alleviate chance are randomisation and large sample sizes. Chance is not an issue in qualitative research, as qualitative research has smaller sample sizes and by nature is not concerned with statistical principles. So in examining a study for flaws due to chance, and depending on the type of study, it is important to look for large sample size, small confidence intervals and be wary of abnormally high or abnormally low results.

In addition, as discussed above, confounders are a common source of flaws in quantitative research. Confounders make it difficult to distinguish whether or not the reported results are a product of several factors at work, rather than the relationship being tested. Confounders can lead to confused and confusing results, which as the appraiser, you must point out. Lastly, the final common flaw that is important to for both quantitative and qualitative research is the lack of rigour.

Barbour (2001, page 115) argues that, especially in terms of qualitative research, ensuring rigour is more than 'technical fixes', such as a prescriptive sampling framework or coding system, but is ensured by 'the systematic and thorough' application of the research methods. Rigour is an overarching concept concerned with the way in which the research is carried out, and how truthfully and conscientiously this is done. If step or stages of the research process are missing or poorly executed, this will have obvious implications on the study's findings, and therefore, as the appraiser, it is important to note if or when the research is lacking in rigour. You will not see a researcher declare, 'this research was conducted unrigorously', and this is up to you as the appraiser to decide.

It is important to notice when judging the rigour of both quantitative and qualitative research that it is as much about the application of the study methodology as it is about the processes followed by the researcher(s). If a study fails to adhere to the principles of the methodology completely or occasionally veers, there are implications for the rigour of the research and potentially the findings.

Before making up your mind about the quality of a study it might be useful to see how others have responded to the research. Makela and Witt (2005) recommend going back to the online version of the article and looking for responses from other readers, which journals sometimes publish shortly after the publication of an article. They suggest that comparing your conclusions with the comments of other readers might provide useful insight.

Once you have reached your decision regarding the study's quality, you must complete the evidence-based practice cycle and decide whether or not this information can and should inform or change current practice.

Case study 4.1: The Grading of Recommendations Assessment, Development and Evaluation (GRADE) Working Group

In 2004 the GRADE Working Group published a critical appraisal of six well-known systems for assessing the level and strength of evidence and recommendations for health care practice. This appraisal set out to investigate the common characteristics and sensibility of these various systems for grading evidence and the strength of recommendations produced. Using a panel of 12 reviewers, the working group graded: (1) the American College of Chest Physicians (ACCP); (2) Australian National Health and Medical Research Council (ANHMRC); (3) Oxford Centre for Evidence-Based Medicine (OCEBM); (4) Scottish Intercollegiate Guidelines Network (SIGN); (5) US Preventive Services Task Force (USPSTF); and (6) US Task Force on Community Preventive Services (USTFCPS).

The working group used 12 criteria to ascertain whether the systems were useful in answering various research questions, could be used by professionals, policy makers or patients or provided clear and appropriate guidelines for grading various types of evidence, taking into account not only the strength of the evidence but the recommendations and the strength of the recommendations made based on the evidence provided. The outcome of the appraisal indicated that none of these six approaches to grading the levels of evidence and strength of recommendations adequately addressed all of the important concepts and dimensions necessary for an adequate and appropriate evidence grading system. The appraisal also concluded that judgements about the quality of evidence should be based on a systematic review of the relevant research and that the availability of systematic review evidence does not correspond to high-quality evidence, as even a well-conducted review might include anything from no studies or poor-quality studies with inconsistent results to high-quality studies with consistent results. This finding called into question the placing of systematic reviews at the top level of grading system and suggested the need for closer scrutiny of research evidence despite its proposed level or strength.

In summary, the GRADE Working Group appraisal illustrates the significance of the principles of critical appraisal in revealing both the commonalities and consistencies as well as the discrepancies and flaws in knowledge, an exercise in finding and making sense of using the strongest and most appropriate evidence.

See Atkins, D et al. (2004) Systems for grading the quality of evidence and the strength of recommendations I: Critical appraisal of existing approaches The GRADE Working Group. *BMC Health Services Research*, 4: 38. Available at: www.biomedcentral.com/1472-6963/4/38

Chapter summary

In summary, critical appraisal is not necessarily about fault finding, but taking note of what is missing, unclear or needs improvement and deciding if these flaws or limitations impact on the credibility of the study's findings. In judging or appraising the evidence it is important to be critical but not damning, as it is much easier to find flaws in other people's work than to create a methodologically flawless piece of work of your own. Critical appraisal is not an opportunity to 'simply rubbish other people's work' but is necessary to make an important judgement about the soundness of evidence provided by the study. It is also important to remember that just because a study is published does not mean that it is flawless, and the job of a critical appraiser is to find the limitations and omissions. A good piece of research will be aware of and declare or attempt to eradicate and/or minimise its limitations.

As mentioned above, all studies are likely to fall short of perfection and it is important to realise this. Studies should be appraised in the light of what they have been able to achieve – they will have deficiencies but, given the particular circumstances, could they realistically have been improved? The evidence they provide may not be strong but, if it is the best that is likely to be available, you should not immediately discount it because of the flaws, but should draw from it what information you can. Likewise, in making your decision about the soundness of the research, you must be cautious, even-handed and logical in your assessment of the study and in formulating your critiques.

As part of the evidence-based practice cycle, your critiques should also be supported with evidence from other research, methodological literature or clinical expertise and justified based on what is presented in the article or study report. If the study reporting provides incomplete or inconclusive information, you ultimately must use and develop the necessary skills to help you decide. Finally, critical appraisal is both the act of judging, but also an art form as it requires you to examine a study as individual parts as well as a whole, and to craft balanced, structured and relevant critiques. The act/art of appraising research may seem like learning to juggle, no easy feat for those of us with poor hand–eye coordination, but it does become easier with practice and with more practice the value for public health practice is continually affirmed.

GOING FURTHER

As this chapter may be your first introduction to critical appraisal, further reading around the area and searching for examples of appraisals is recommended.
Below is a list of useful websites, some of which include critical appraisal tools, tutorials, course information or worked examples. This is by no means an exhaustive list, but a good starting point.

- University of Oxford Centre for Evidence Based Medicine: www.cebm.net/
- Superego Cafe: www.criticalappraisal.com/
- University of Kent: www.kent.ac.uk/library/subjects/healthinfo/critapprais. html
- Solutions for Public Health Unit: www.sph.nhs.uk/what-we-do/public-health-workforce/resources/critical-appraisals-skills-programme
- University of the West of England: http://hsc.uwe.ac.uk/dataanalysis/ critIntro.asp
- Scottish Intercollegiate Guidelines Network (SIGN): www.sign.ac.uk/ methodology/checklists.html
- London Journal of Primary Care Checklists: www.londonjournalofprimarycare. org/checklists/

chapter 5

Assessing Evidence – the Quality of Primary and Secondary Research
Amina Dilmohamed and Mahwish Hayee

Meeting the public health competences

Core area 2: Assessing the evidence of effectiveness of interventions, programmes and services to improve population health and wellbeing.

This chapter will help you to evidence the following competences for public health (Public Health Skills and Careers Framework):

- Level 6 (b) Knowledge of the principles of critical appraisal as applied to various studies, and its use in improving health and wellbeing
- Level 6 (c) Understanding of the levels of evidence and their importance for decision-making in own area of work
- Level 7 (a) Understanding of appraising the quality of primary and secondary research
- Level 7 (b) Understanding of the hierarchy of evidence as it applies to services, programmes and interventions which impact on health and wellbeing
- Level 8 (1) Make and influence decisions based on evidence of effectiveness
- Level 8 (2) Challenge the decisions that others make when evidence has not been taken into account.

This chapter will also assist you in demonstrating the following National Occupational Standard(s) for public health:

- Reflect on and develop your practice – (HSC33)
- Support and challenge workers on specific aspects of their practice – (CJ F309)
- Develop evidence based clinical guidelines – (HI127)
- Create and capitalise upon opportunities to advocate the need for improving health and wellbeing – (PHP46)
- Communicate effectively with the public and others about improving the health and wellbeing of the population – (PHS11).

This chapter will also be useful in demonstrating Standards 4c and 4e and 7 of the Public Health Practitioner Standards:

- Standard 4. Continually develop and improve own and others' practice in public health by:

    d. the application of evidence in improving own area of work
    e. objectively and constructively contributing to reviewing the effectiveness of own area of work.

- Standard 7. Assess the evidence of effective interventions and services to improve health and wellbeing – demonstrating:

   a. knowledge of the different types, sources and levels of evidence in own area of practice and how to access and use them
   b. the appraisal of published evidence and the identification of implications for own area of work practice.

Chapter overview

The purpose of this chapter is to address the methods in which both primary and secondary research can be assessed for its quality. As the lack of consensus on the specific standards for assessing quality research and standards of quality for assessing evidence are debatable (Gersten et al., 2000; Mosteller and Boruch, 2002) and several researchers have contended that some of the current peer-review processes and standards for assessing quality are not well suited for research in specific areas (Gersten et al., 2000; NCDDR, 2003; Spooner and Browder, 2003).

Public health interventions tend to be complex; therefore the evidence for their effectiveness must be sufficiently comprehensive to encompass that complexity. Therefore we need to address 'quality' and 'evidence' as separate entities. So, research quality can be seen as the scientific process, evidence quality pertains more to a judgement regarding the strength and confidence found in the research which emanates from the scientific process (Mosteller and Boruch, 2002; Shavelson and Towne, 2002).

Why should research quality be assessed?

The very idea of evidence-based public health rests on remarkably brave claims that evidence should have a privileged voice in public health practice because there are objective methods available to judge and justify the quality of the advice provided by public health (medical) research. These objective measures, called the 'evidence hierarchies', have become common notions of evidence assessment ever since they were introduced by two American social scientists in the 1960s.

So why bother with assessing or judging the quality of evidence? History shows that if research quality is assessed before adopting it in clinical practice or in health policy it helps in many ways. Some of these advantages will be considered here. The first is that it helps to protect against errors; second it helps to resolve disagreements and when the quality of studies is rigorously assessed before adopting them into practice they go through systematic critical appraisal during this process. After quality assessment the information is usually disseminated in an easily communicable way.

Scenario

Consider the following and how you would address the issues relating to nursing interventions in the effective management of COPD (chronic obstructive pulmonary disease). In the field of public health large-scale intervention is generally the norm, therefore assessing the quality of research is paramount in guiding a positive outcome. This scenario will indicate the importance of assessing literature and how the findings impact on health practices.

William is a 55-year-old retired builder who has been coughing constantly during the last two weeks before he was brought to the hospital by his youngest daughter. Lately, he has been experiencing troubles in breathing. He described it as a difficulty in expiration during breathing. For this reason, he asked his youngest daughter who is living just two blocks away from him to take him to the hospital.

William admits to being a chronic smoker, consuming two packs per day and drinks alcoholic beverages regularly with his friends. After undergoing a thorough examination, his physician ordered a series of sputum tests and other lung tests. Chronic infection was detected in the lungs, most probably due to smoking, which irritates the bronchi and bronchioles. There was also obstruction of the airways which is responsible for the patient's difficulty in expiration. He was diagnosed with COPD.

Problem diagnosis/description

The chronic infection is caused by the patient's excessive smoking or other substances which irritate the bronchi and the bronchioles. The principal reason for the chronic infection is that the irritant seriously disrupts the normal protective mechanisms of the airways, the effects of nicotine causing partial paralysis of the cilia of the respiratory epithelium. As a result, mucus cannot be moved easily out of the passageways (Guyton and Hall, 2000).

Nursing diagnosis reveals ineffective airway clearance related to excessive and tenacious secretions. The assessment criteria include William's ability to maintain an upright position, cough and sputum. Diagnosis further reveals activity intolerance related to fatigue and inadequate oxygenation. Assessment criteria include tolerance to activities of daily living and aggravating factors. Another nursing diagnosis is anxiety related to breathlessness and fear of suffocation. Assessment criteria include William's anxiety level and his knowledge of breathing techniques.

Other possible nursing diagnoses for William include: (1) powerlessness related to feeling of loss of control and the restrictions that this condition places on his lifestyle; (2) sleep pattern disturbance related to cough, inability to assume recumbent position and environmental stimuli; and (3) high risk for altered nutrition: which is less than body requirements related to anorexia and secondary to dyspnoea, halitosis and fatigue.

Possible nursing interventions you may consider when searching literature

Interventions for ineffective airway clearance include: (1) teaching William the proper controlled coughing methods; (2) teaching him methods to reduce the viscosity of the cough secretions; and (3) auscultation of the lungs prior to and after coughing exercises. Uncontrolled coughing is ineffective and would tend to make William feel frustrated, therefore it is important to teach him controlled coughing methods. Because thick secretions, which are difficult to expectorate, can cause mucus plugs, leading to atelectasis, the patient needs to be taught methods to reduce the viscosity of secretions. Auscultation can help to evaluate the effectiveness of coughing exercises.

Nursing interventions for activity intolerance related to fatigue and inadequate oxygenation for activities include: (1) explaining to William the factors that increase oxygen demand, which in turn can cause an increased cardiac workload and oxygen requirements; (2) teaching the patient methods of conserving energy, which can then help prevent excessive energy expenditure; (3) increasing the patient's activity as tolerated since moderate breathlessness improves accessory muscle strength; (4) maintaining supplemental oxygen therapy which can increase circulating oxygen levels and improve tolerance; and (5) post-activity assessment for abnormal responses to activity increase and monitoring for decreased pulse, decreased or unchanged systolic blood pressure, and excessively increased or decreased respirations.

Nursing interventions for William's anxiety related to breathlessness and fear of suffocation include: (1) providing a calm, quiet environment when the patient is experiencing episodes of breathlessness which can promote relaxation; (2) not leaving the patient alone or unattended when he is experiencing episodes of breathlessness; and (3) helping the patient with all his tasks during acute episodes since during this time he will be unable to perform activities that he usually does.
Individuals with a family history of lung disease and those with an early onset of emphysema should be tested for α_1-antitrypsin deficiency to determine serum levels. Phenotyping should be done if the level is low.

The normal phenotype is constituted by the MM genetic pattern. The most common abnormal phenotype associated with α_1-antitrypsin deficiency is the ZZ pattern. Individuals with the MZ phenotype are carriers of the disease, but do not appear to have an increased risk of developing COPD (Boyle and Locke, 2004).

William has to undergo COPD therapy. He also has to quit smoking and drinking for it will be futile to undergo therapy and still continue with his health-damaging habits. He should be constantly monitored by the nurses and by his daughter as well so that his therapy will be effective.

(Adapted with permission from: casestudiessamples. blogspot.com/.../sample-nursing-copd-case-study.html)

Reflection

William's case is not hopeless. Chronic obstructive pulmonary diseases are experienced by many individuals worldwide. There are many drugs that can help patients who have COPD. But of course, these drugs alone cannot cure the ailment.

In this case the patient has to stop his smoking and drinking habits as this will only worsen his condition. Smoking will eventually destroy his lungs even if he is taking drugs that are used in COPD therapy.

Appropriate care (both pharmacological and pulmonary rehabilitation) according to guidelines can relieve symptoms, improve quality of life and reduce exacerbation rates (NICE, 2004). The MRC dyspnoea score reflects functional status (Bestall *et al.*, 1999) and can alert clinicians to the increasing clinical and social needs.

ACTIVITY 5.1

After reading the scenario above and familiarising yourself with the medical terminology, follow the step-by-step process to assist you in understanding why finding the most appropriate research is key in answering questions.

Step 1: Asking the question

Examples: questions can be related to diagnosis, treatment, quality or economics. Questions should be *specific* and must take into account:

- The type of patient
- The nature of the intervention(s)
- The desired outcome.

Step 2: Finding the evidence

In the context of evidence-based practice there are two main sources of evidence:

- Bibliographic databases (e.g. CINAHL, MEDLINE)
- Publication-based databases (e.g. the Cochrane Database of Systematic Reviews) (see Chapter 2 for more databases).

Step 3: Appraising the evidence

The questions that need to be asked are:

- What are the results and findings?
- Are the results valid?
- Will the results impact on the care of the patient or population?

Step 4: Acting on the evidence

- Changing practice according to the evidence
- Developing new policies.

Step 5: Evaluation

- Has the change worked for this situation?

The following examples will give you an idea of what we are endeavouring to aim for when conducting and assessing evidence relevant to practice. You will notice that each example has only been given one source of evidence.

ACTIVITY 5.2

You are asked to search for further evidence to support the following scenario issues by following the step-by-step process to find the most relevant research to answer the questions in the individual scenarios.

Scenario 1

Mr Daniels is a 35-year-old father with two young children, who recently lost his wife in a road accident. He has been suffering from depression and his family are very concerned about him. He was very active until the death of his wife; the family used to enjoy long walks and he exercised at the local gym three times a week.

- **Question:** Will exercise be helpful in treating his depression?

- **Evidence**: Lane, AM and Lovejoy, DJ (2001) The effects of exercise on mood changes: the moderating effect of depressed mood. *Journal of Sports Medicine and Physical Fitness* 41(4): 539–545. The study is a randomised controlled trial to assess the effects of exercise on negative mood.
- **Results**: The findings of this study found the reduction in anger, confusion, fatigue, tension and vigour was significantly greater in the depressed mood group who had undergone exercise therapy.

Scenario 2

Mr Khan is a 45-year-old South Indian Asian who has three sons, Salim being the youngest. Salim attends the local primary school. On Tuesday morning after assembly he was taken to hospital and admitted to the children's ward and diagnosed with type 1 diabetes. Needless to say Salim was distraught.

- **Question**: Would Salim benefit from home care or hospital care?
- **Evidence**: Dougherty, G, Schiffrin, A and White, D (1999) Home based management can achieve intensification cost effectively in type 1 diabetes. *Paediatrics* 103: 122–128.
- **Results**: This is a randomised control trial with three years follow-up involving 63 children. Children managed with home-based care had improved glycaemic control and similar knowledge and compliance with treatment.

What is the meaning of quality of evidence?

Let us define what we mean by 'quality of evidence' in the context of making recommendations. The quality of evidence reflects the extent to which our confidence in an estimate of the effect is adequate to support a particular recommendation. In the context of a systematic review the quality of evidence reflects the extent to which we are confident that an estimate of effect is correct.

Before venturing off to discuss the details of quality of evidence it will be beneficial to explain its meaning to the readers of this book. Quality of evidence is defined as: 'the quality of evidence indicates the extent to which one can be confident that an estimate of effect is correct. The strength of a recommendation indicates the extent to which one can be confident that adherence to the recommendation will do more good than harm' (Schünemann *et al.*, 2008).

Now if you are wondering what the estimate of effect means then it will be explained in this paragraph. If we look at effect size in the perspective of statistics it simply means that it is a measure of the strength of relationship between two variables in a statistically selected population (this is mostly a random sample taken from the population). To take a simple example, if we are studying weight loss in children and the programme reports a weight loss of 10 pounds, then the 10 pounds is an indicator of the effect size.

In medical practice, clinicians often try to look for a single piece of information which they can incorporate in their practice. This information could be the effect of a treatment, the information provided by a diagnostic test or the effect of a harmful exposure. Studies generally report point estimates of effects. The point estimates of effects from different studies may differ widely and it would be very difficult to have to look at a whole range of studies when deciding promptly what treatment approach to adopt. Therefore, the quantitative systematic review, also called meta-analysis, provides a single best summary of estimate of effect. To do this results are statistically combined by reviewers of meta-analysis. This is a very rigorous process and the quality of these studies is assessed by applying stringent criteria.

Primary and secondary research designs

Research designs can be broadly divided into primary and secondary research. In primary research, data is collected from, for example, research subjects or experiments. To explain it further, primary research is carried out when the researchers collect data for the area that they are researching by themselves. In most cases this data did not previously exist. In academic language this is also sometimes referred to as empirical research. Data collection for this purpose can be done by using qualitative or quantitative approaches (Table 5.1).

Table 5.1 Primary research methods

Qualitative	Quantitative
Focus groups	Surveys • Personal interviews • Telephone, fax, email • In-house self-administered • Mail
In-depth interviews Observation studies	Experiments

Secondary research involves the summary, collation and/or synthesis of existing research rather than primary research, where data is collected from, for example, research subjects or experiments (Crouch *et al.*, 2003). The data are already collected and available for the researchers to analyse. Alternatively, studies that have been published are analysed to come up with an answer to a research question. In public health research the most common way of reporting the data after its rigorous quality assessment is systematic review. Systematic reviews may or may not have a quantitative element to them. When the quantitative part is included then it is called a meta-analysis, as mentioned earlier in the chapter.

Secondary research

Secondary research is where one uses information that other people have gathered through primary research. The next obvious question would be, why do we use secondary research? Well because it has its advantages, it is inexpensive, easily accessible, immediately available, will provide essential background and help to clarify or refine research problem essential for literature review. Secondary data sources will provide research method alternatives and will also alert the researcher to any potential difficulties. Like all good things there are some disadvantages of secondary research. Studies are frequently outdated, for example sample data, potentially unreliable, you are not always sure where information has come from and it may not be applicable, may not totally answer your research questions, lack of availability (i.e. no data available or very difficult to obtain).

Locating secondary source

- Bibliographies (are compiled lists of sources on a particular subject)
- Books (online library catalogue)
- Articles (that interpret or review research works).

How can I tell if something is a secondary source?

As with any research, examine the document or article carefully for accuracy and credibility. Use the following questions to help you determine whether or not you are using a credible secondary source.

Authors

- How does the author know what he/she knows?
- Does his/her knowledge stem from personal experience or having read about and analysed an event?
- Does the author cite several other (published) reports?

Content

- Why is the information being provided or the article written?
- Are there references to other writings on this topic?
- Is the author interpreting previous events?
- Does the information come from personal experience or others' accounts?

Currency/timeliness

- Is the date of publication evident?
- Is the date of publication close to the event described or was it written much later?

Current GRADE approaches for quality of evidence

Too many systems

There is a bewildering variety of systems to rate the quality of evidence underlying recommendations and guidelines. Developers are inconsistent with how they rate this evidence. Listed below are five independent bodies that support the development of evidence-based national clinical guidelines and facilitate their implementation into practice for the benefit of patients. Their aim is to ensure appropriate involvement of healthcare professionals, patients and carers; unfortunately no generic standard has been employed, therefore failing to develop a process to create internationally agreed standards of guideline.

- US Preventative Services Task Force
- Scottish Intercollegiate Guidelines (SIGN)
- Australian National Health and Medical Research Council
- Oxford Centre for Evidence-Based Medicine
- Professional organisations.

As a result, users have faced challenges. GRADE offers a systematic method of assessing the quality of studies included in a systematic review and developing recommendations or guidelines based upon the evidence. Its aim is to develop a common, transparent and sensible system for grading the quality of evidence and the strength of recommendations.

The following organisations have adopted the GRADE system:

- Agency for Health Care Research and Quality (AHRQ)
- Allergic Rhinitis in Asthma Guidelines (ARIA)
- American College of Chest Physicians
- American College of Physicians
- American Thoracic Society
- British Medical Journal
- Canadian Agency for Drugs and Technology in Health
- Clinical Evidence

- Cochrane Collaboration

- European Society of Thoracic Surgeons

- Infectious Diseases Society of America (IDSA)

- National Institute for Health and Clinical Excellence (NICE)

- UpToDate

- World Health Organization.

Determinants of quality

How do we then determine the quality of research? We generally appreciate that study design is critical to judgements about the quality of evidence and that randomised trials provide stronger evidence than observational studies and that, furthermore, observational studies provide stronger evidence than uncontrolled case series.

The GRADE approach to quality

Under the GRADE system, quality of evidence is accepted when randomised trials without important limitations provide high-quality evidence. Observational studies without special strengths provide low-quality evidence. Limitations or special strengths may modify the quality of the evidence of both randomised trials and observational studies.

The GRADE system classifies the quality of evidence according to four grades:

- Very low – this makes for very uncertain estimates of effect.

- Low – quantifying the effect is still uncertain and is highly likely to be changed by further research.

- Moderate – further research is likely to significantly change the degree of confidence which can be attached to the estimate of effects.

- High – further research is very unlikely to change the degree of confidence in the estimate of effect.

GRADE have also developed a software programme called 'GradePro'. This provides information on three types of evidence:

- GRADE evidence profile

- Cochrane Summary of Findings (SoF) table (SoF table is the most useful for most Cochrane reviews)

- Cochrane Overview of Reviews table.

GRADE evidence profile

These are particularly useful for guideline developers. They present information about the body of evidence (e.g. number of studies), the judgements about the underlying quality of evidence, key statistical results, and a grade for the quality of evidence for each outcome. They are more instructive than SoF tables.

Summary of findings

These are most relevant to (and designed for use in) Cochrane reviews. They present the main findings of a systematic review in a transparent and simple tabular format. They provides key information concerning the quality of evidence, the magnitude of effect of the interventions examined, and the sum of available data on most important outcomes.

Case study 5.1: Do pedometers increase physical activity in sedentary older women? A randomized controlled trial

Objectives: To determine the effectiveness of a behaviour change intervention (BCI) with or without a pedometer in increasing physical activity in sedentary older women.

Design: Prospective randomised controlled trial.

Setting: Primary care, City of Dundee, Scotland.

Participants: Two hundred and four sedentary women aged 70 and older.

Interventions: Six months of BCI, BCI plus pedometer (pedometer plus), or usual care.

Measurements: Primary outcome: change in daily activity counts measured by accelerometry. Secondary outcomes: Short Physical Performance Battery; health-related quality of life; depression and anxiety; falls; National Health Service resource use.

Results: Eighty-eight per cent (179 of 204) women completed the six-month trial. Withdrawals were highest from the BCI group (15/68) followed by the pedometer plus group (8/68) and then the control group (2/64). After adjustment for baseline differences, accelerometry counts increased significantly more in the BCI group at three months than in the control group ($P = 0.002$) and the pedometer plus group ($P = 0.04$). By six months, accelerometry counts in both intervention groups had fallen to levels that were no longer statistically significantly different from baseline. There were no significant changes in the secondary outcomes.

Conclusion: The BCI was effective in objectively increasing physical activity in sedentary older women. Provision of a pedometer yielded no additional benefit in physical activity, but may have motivated participants to remain in the trial.

ACTIVITY 5.3

After reading the case study:

- Use the GRADE approach to assess the quality of this case study.
- How do rank this study?
- Justify your choice.
- Spend a few minutes thinking about these questions and write down your answers.

Chapter summary

This chapter started with how primary and secondary research could be assessed for quality. It further revealed that guidelines developers globally were seen to be inconsistent on how they rate quality of evidence and grade strength of recommendation which created a gap as there was no generic format of assessing quality. In order to facilitate learning we introduced you to 'GRADE' (Grading of Recommendations Assessment, Development and Evaluation). This system of evidence is used when submitting to clinical guideline article. We then took you through a step-by-step process on how to answer a research question; this concise method aimed to draw to your attention how to make it easier to identify relevant and appropriate research for the question posed.

The key features of this chapter are:

- The importance of assessing evidence

- Where to access the evidence

- What tool/method should be used in deciding the quality of evidence found

- Disseminating the evidence and its effects on public health.

- GRADE Working Group www.gradeworkinggroup.org
  The Grading of Recommendations Assessment, Development and Evaluation (GRADE) Working Group began in the year 2000 as an informal collaboration of people with an interest in addressing the shortcomings of present grading systems in health care. The working group has developed a common, sensible and transparent approach to grading quality of evidence and strength of recommendations.

chapter 6

Assessing Evidence – the Strengths and Weaknesses of Various Ways of Assessing Public Health Outcomes

Krishna Regmi

Meeting the public health competences

Core area 2: Assessing the evidence of effectiveness of interventions, programmes and services to improve population health and wellbeing.

This chapter will help you to evidence the following competences for public health (Public Health Skills and Careers Framework):

- Level 6 (b) Knowledge of the principles of critical appraisal as applied to various studies, and its use in improving health and wellbeing
- Level 7 (c) Understanding of the strengths and weaknesses of various ways of assessing outcomes.

This chapter will also assist you in demonstrating the following National Occupational Standard(s) for public health:

- Assess the evidence and impact of health and healthcare – (PHS07) interventions, programmes and services and apply the assessments to practice
- Improve the quality of health and healthcare interventions and services through audit and evaluation – (PHS08)
- Monitor and review effectiveness of services and initiatives to protect health, wellbeing and safety – (HP10)
- Support and challenge workers on specific aspects of their practice – (CJ F309).

This chapter will also be useful in demonstrating Standard 7 of the Public Health Practitioner Standards:

- Standard 7. Assess the evidence of effective interventions and services to improve health and wellbeing – demonstrating:

a. knowledge of the different types, sources and levels of evidence in own area of practice and how to access and use them
b. the appraisal of published evidence and the identification of implications for own area of work practice.

Chapter overview

The concept of evidence has been thoroughly debated within the medical literature as the meaning and interpretation of 'evidence' has varied among different academic and professional fields. Recently, the evidence-based approach has emerged in many disciplines, including medicine, public health, nursing, social care, health policy and other allied healthcare, as well as non-healthcare, sectors. Trinder and Reynolds (2000, page 3) argue that the notion of using evidence-based practice is 'self-evidently a good idea', and the practice is often effective because it is based on the 'most up-to-date, valid and reliable' evidence (see also Green, 1999). But is that often the case? And to what extent is this assertion valid in terms of producing a reliable outcome? This chapter will discuss these questions.

Exercises in this chapter will focus on:

- developing clarity about the meaning of 'evidence' in public health;
- being aware of the tools and techniques to assess the outcomes of evidence in evidence-based practice; and
- examining the problems in assessing any public health outcomes.

Learning outcomes

After reading this chapter you will be able to:

- critically discuss what is meant by evidence and how to assess evidence in public health and wellbeing;
- critically discuss what factors influence assessment and evaluation of evidence-based practice/implementation;
- discuss different methods of assessing evidence in terms of quality, and examine their strengths and weaknesses.

Introduction

This chapter discusses the assessment of assessing evidence and the nature and types of assessment, and examines the strengths and weakness of different approaches/methods when assessing public health outcomes. Although the definition of evidence-based medicine has been widely used in health and social care, different professionals conceptualise its terms differently. Sheldon and Chilvers (2000, page 5) define evidence-based medicine as the 'conscientious, explicit and judicious use of current best evidence in making decisions about the care of individual patients based on skills which allow the doctor to evaluate both personal experience and external evidence in a systematic and objective manner' (adapted from Sackett *et al.*, 1996). In Sackett *et al.*'s (2000, page 5 and see also Ilic, 2009, page 1) view, evidence-based medicine means 'making decisions informed by most relevant and valid evidence available'. From this concept, one can easily argue that there are different aspects involved in making decisions, for example, knowledge, attitude, practice and behaviour of both decision makers and policy planners. Therefore, Naidoo and Wills (forthcoming) argue that the role of evidence-based medicine in public health is complex. Public health embeds a number of different multifactorial aspects in interventions to improve population health and wellbeing. For example, strategies for reducing health inequality include education, providing health service access to poor and disadvantaged groups, and changing policy on an inclusive welfare society. Therefore it is difficult to claim which strategies are the most effective. As Naidoo and Wills claim, these strategies might not be universally employed as these may vary in different areas in practice. In some cases, there might be a robust piece of evidence to demonstrate the effectiveness of such strategies, but because there is either a lack of practitioners' awareness, easily accessible resources or capacity, or because it is inappropriate to the given circumstances, practices may be slow to change.

ACTIVITY 6.1

Reflection: Can you share your understanding or interpretation of evidence-based practice? List at least three advantages and three disadvantages of evidence-based practice.

Comment: Some of the advantages you identified might have included being confident that practice is based on knowing what works and that the planned public health intervention is likely to provide the intended outcomes. Having a clear understanding of the evidence base for public health practice is useful but is not always easy to do. It takes time and in public health is complex. However, basing practice on a firm evidence base can help to ensure that it is more effective. If the evidence exists then it is easier to solve the problem, planning becomes easier and where evidence underpins practice it is more likely that it will deliver the intended health outcomes.

Assessment and evaluation of public health outcomes

The World Health Organization (2003, pages 3–4) notes that in many developed and developing nations there are five common problems in assessing any public health outcomes. First, the design of public health services is often complicated, which leads to a lack of clarity about the nature of fundamental goals. Furthermore, national health policy is often focused on short-term objectives or on instrumental goals such as cost containment, expanding public infrastructure, reducing patient waiting times for consultation or introducing user fees, and consequently often lose sight of the primary goal of the health system – improving public health and wellbeing. Second, policy planners and decision makers often consult on the issue of health services design with someone whom they trust; the answer substantially depends upon which expert is asked, and the response may vary depending upon the nature and background of the consultations. Third, in many public health interventions, health systems are fragmented, and the stakeholders are only concerned with certain factors at any one time. For example, decision makers are only accountable to the resources and activity, whereas government may be responsible for improving health and wellbeing across the population. Fourth, in many public health interventions the remit of strategic focus has been directed towards 'delivering certain proven technology' (page 4) such as vaccinations or Directly Observed Short-Course Therapy (DOTS) for tuberculosis. It has been claimed that cost-effective strategies to improve public health outcomes are an important aspect of public health policy, but such policy lacks, for example, developing human health capacity, health service provision or inclusive health programmes (WHO, 2003). Therefore it can be argued that devising an inclusive and balanced strategy while dealing with public health issues or outcomes might be warranted. Finally, a public health system is complex, and has many interactive determinants, including specialised language. Such complexities create barriers to prevent wider public participation in the health policy debate. WHO (2003) therefore strongly advocates that assessing pubic health means 'empowering civil society and the general public to become active participants' in the formulation of national and local health policies (page 5). Gray (1997, cited in Jenkinson, 1997, page 2) argues that patients' decisions are made on the basis of 'patients' personal values, available resources and evidence'.

Decisions in health care and public health are still made based on the personal values and available resources, with little consideration of the importance of evidence. However, there is a gradual recognition of the importance of evidence being realised in making any public health decisions. Das *et al.* (2008, page 493) argue that the role of evidence-based medicine (EBM) has become increasingly popular in the NHS in terms of resource allocation, delivery and provision of health care policy and research (also see NHS, 1996) and, this is also evident in wider public health. Jenkinson (1997) warns that any assessment or evaluation should be both critical and objective in manner.

ACTIVITY 6.2

Reflection: What are the common problems in assessing any public health outcomes? How should they be addressed?

Comment: You may have identified the sheer complexity of any public health intervention and the associated difficulty of being sure that an outcome is solely a result of the public health programme as a key problem in assessing public health outcomes. So many other variables are likely to be involved. These problems can be partially addressed by being clear about the outcomes that a public health programme is trying to achieve. Using a clear public health planning framework and identifying key outcomes to be monitored from the outset can make the process more straightforward.

Often assessments of public health outcomes are based on the individual's experience and clinical anecdotes (Holland, 1983). Evaluation means determining which intervention (e.g. treatment) is the most effective, and which should be continued (Jenkinson, 1997). Rossi and Freeman (1985) argue that in any assessment or evaluation, the following activities are often interconnected:

- 'Analysing related to the conceptualisation and the design of the invention',

- 'Monitoring of programme implementation' and

- 'Assessment of programme utility' (page 380).

Process, approach and methods of assessing evidence

'Evaluation may be defined as a careful and critical analysis of a situation leading to the drawing of sensible conclusions and making purposeful proposals for future action' (Mella *et al.*, 2000, page 296).

Evaluation or assessment is thus a basic function of management. From the very start, in deciding on public health programmes or interventions, we are involved in assessment. As the programme or intervention is carried out, continuous assessment (monitoring) and evaluation will be performed to see if there are problems in the implementation, and if feasible solutions to these problems can be proposed. This might be similar to the notion of continuous quality improvement (CQI). At the end of the intervention, assessment is done to see whether the set of desired outcomes at the beginning were met. Mella *et al.* (2000) argued that assessment therefore is a 'continuous process and never stops' (page 295). The results of assessments are fed back into the planning process again. Assessment therefore is a non-linear process occurring in all phases of the health management cycle: planning, deciding what intervention(s) to implement, implementation and post-implementation (follow-up). This means that there are many types of assessment or evaluation, with each type undertaken depending upon the purpose for which assessment is done.

Ewles and Simnett set out a framework for planning and evaluating health promotion (Figure 6.1) which builds on this notion of continuous improvement. They identify 9 steps (or stages) including identifying clients, identifying client needs and determining goals for health education which are then refined into specific objectives. Resources are identified and more detailed planning of the health education programme takes place. Evaluation methods are planned and the health education programme carried out and evaluated. Importantly, for each of the nine steps in the framework there is a feedback loop.

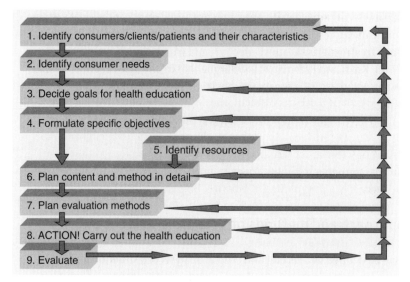

Figure 6.1 Planning and evaluating health promotion framework.

Source: Adapted from Ewles and Simnett (2010, page 65). Reproduced with permission.

ACTIVITY 6.3

Reflection: 'Evaluation may be defined as a careful and critical analysis of a situation leading to the drawing of sensible conclusions and making purposeful proposals for future action' (Mella *et al.*, 2000, page 296). How far do you agree or disagree with this definition, and why?

Comment: You may have agreed that many health education programmes are clear about the target group and their identified needs and have clear overall goals. Objectives are often very specific and clearly stated but this is not always the case. Resources may be clearly identified and adequate resources may be available but in many instances the identified resources may be inadequate or only available in the short term. Clear planning of the content and delivery of the health education often gets the most attention. In some programmes the evaluation is not given sufficient attention at this stage. In some programmes, this step is often left until the end of the programme, and is planned and undertaken, after the health education has been undertaken. Building in evaluation and evaluating the intervention from the outset can provide some leverage to argue for the longer-term implementation of the programme.

You might have identified the need to consider short-term indicators and measures of success, particularly in step 8, or even have suggested that there should be mini-evaluation cycles built into each stage,

Nature and types of assessment and evaluation

Although people often use the term assessment and evaluation interchangeably in different contexts, it may be useful to be familiar with these concepts. Assessment is defined as a process to determine whether or not intended outcomes are being achieved whereas evaluation uses assessment information in making appropriate decisions in practice (Gagne *et al.*, 1998). Commonly, measurements/achievements are categorised in terms of whether they focus on the process (assessment) or on the outcomes (evaluation). In Dahlberg and McCaig's view (2010, page16) assessment often links with the strengths and weaknesses in a programme while evaluation aims to measure the success of a programme in practice. Both assessment and evaluation inform policy planners and decision makers on how to improve the services effectively. Often assessment is interpreted in terms of summative feedback, while evaluation might be considered more summative formative in nature, which is not always the case. Assessment, however, is one of the young disciplines in management science, and the nature of evaluation is often 'vast, lumbering, overgrown' (Pawson and Tilley, 1997, page 1). Sometimes it is difficult to assess where we are now, where we can go, with whom, why and how, etc. In Kaplan's (1964, cited in Pawson and Tilley, 1997, page 1) view, evaluation can be considered with the term of 'law of hammer' to discover the universal truth that 'everything needs pounding'.

Chelimsky (1995) highlights some critical links between evaluation and its roles in making decisions. She suggests three key roles for evaluation: first, to avoid reinventing the wheel, second, to provide timely monitoring and third, to establish the outcomes of initiatives. She also acknowledges that evaluation is not an easy task, sometimes bringing some unintended or unwanted messages. She therefore suggests that the reported findings should be based on evidence using the principles of independently verified, appropriate criticism and balance.

Abrams (1995) argues that assessing simply means what does work for whom in what context that is echoed by the equation of Pawson and Tilley (1997, page xv): 'Mechanism + Context = Outcomes'. The nation of this equation is that 'outcomes follow from mechanisms acting in context' (page 58). As Pawson and Tilley discuss, the mechanism considers some aspects of 'choices and capacities' within the context of public health problems. This approach, for example, examines the viewpoint of 'why' some interventions work and some do not. The meaning and interpretation of 'context' here is very much the interventions, for example, which public health problem mechanisms are activated, and in which programme mechanisms (interventions) can be successfully implemented. This approach links to a better understanding of 'for whom and in what circumstances a public health programme works through the study of contextual conditioning' (page 216). Public health is complex in nature, and includes multiple mechanisms in multiple contexts, therefore assessing evidence requires assessing and identifying the people and the situations for whom the particular public health intervention would be effective, by examining the risks and benefits within and between interventions (page 217). The final element of Pawson and Tilley's equation is the 'outcomes'. It has been argued that to assess the outcomes, researchers need to examine and understand what the outcomes of a particular public health intervention are, and how they are achieved (Pawson and Tilley,

1997, page 217). Outcomes are considered a key evidence to monitor and modify any health programmes. As any health interventions have multiple mechanisms, it can be argued that they offer multiple health outcomes, therefore outcomes cannot be linked whether this is an evidence of work, but this should be viewed from the perspective of whether this is the outcome of the combination of mechanism and/or context (Pawson and Tilley, 1997).

Assessing outcomes

Outcomes can be assessed in different ways in different contexts and different disciplines, either qualitative, quantitative or a combination of both methods. Although there are no clear-cut divisions between qualitative and quantitative approaches, and they are not mutually exclusive, the quantitative approach aims to measure and quantify facts and their relationships, seeking to understand these relationships through statistical analysis of data, whereas the qualitative approach usually collects experiences, interpretations, impressions or motivation of an individual or individuals, and as such is characteristically language-based and descriptive rather than analytical (Hennink, 2007; Silverman, 2010). Each method has its own merits and demerits; for example, a quantitative evaluation approach could have provided a more representative view, but would not have provided the depth of understanding allowed by this approach. Therefore Regmi et al. (2010) argue that adopting a combined approach utilising the maximum variation strategy evaluation process would capture the 'focus on diversity' of the issues and concerns of both participants and systems in assessing public health outcomes. Knapp (1996, page 21) argues that assessment or evaluation of any interventions is complex due to 'the nature of collaborative or integrated effort, and convergence of different disciplines'.

Recently, the 'process approach' in assessing and evaluating evidence has been highlighted in public health outcomes, as the process approach involves how something happens rather than examining the final products – outputs and outcomes at the end of the intervention (Patton, 2002). As Patton argues, the notion of process approach is 'what we do is no more important than how we do it' (page 159). This means that people's participation is a key in any public health programme development and implementation process rather than an end in itself, not just a means to some more concrete end; the process is the point, rather than simply the means of arriving at some other point (Patton, 2002). Smith et al. (2005) also note that process evaluation seeks to assess or measure a change in the way that care is provided affects the health of individuals or populations and this approach often intends to compare one form of health care or health intervention with another, or with no care. However in some interventions, for example, biomedical and clinical sciences, the approach plays down the process, meaning that more focus is given to results and outcomes. Patton (2002, page 159), however, strongly argues that even in these cases, 'some process is undertaken to achieve results and understanding the process–outcomes relationship necessitates documenting and understanding the process'.

Although evidence-based practice has been advocated positively, there is little evidence to show the effectiveness of different methods (Hatala and Guyatt, 2002), as assessing evidence is a difficult area to investigate due to the lack of conceptual clarity about the evidence-based medicine or practice itself, and the complexities of analysing processes, especially the attribution of outcomes to particular policies related to public health interventions. Lockett (1997) points out that the effect of evidence-based medicine on health care practice, including public health practice, has been a mixed picture; for example, he noted some positive outcomes of screening procedures, but its effect on patient care is more complex due to the 'lacking of current methodologies to assess outcomes' (page 28). Lockett further noted that Knapp (1996, page 21) points out that the design of any service assessments 'must first accommodate the sheer number of players, stakeholders, and levels of the system as services join forces to influence the lives of people'. Several authors (Sackett *et al.*, 2000; Brown *et al.*, 2006) advocate that a 'PICOT' – patients' intervention, comparison intervention, outcomes and time stamp – approach would be an appropriate framework to assess the evidence. Although some argued that 'PICOT' should be an essential component of research recommendation, still this framework lacks some aspects of contextual elements – state of the evidence, the nature and type of study, and the time factor. Another argument made by Brown *et al.* (2006, page 806) is that such a framework (PICOT) is inappropriate due to 'uncertainties of the effects of any form of health intervention or treatment and is intended for research in humans rather than basic scientific research', therefore the purpose of this format varies among authors, target audiences, and intended purpose and outcomes. Regardless of the criticisms, Del Mar *et al.* (2004) argue that evidence-based medicine allows us to keep health professionals' practice up to date within the complex world of medicine.

Case study 6.1: Different kinds of evidence

There is huge variation in the way the evidence of impact has been sought – from informal discussion at team meetings through to more formal and independent processes of evaluation. Most often articles/reports appear to contain the researchers' reflections on the impact of working with the public on a particular project. In other cases, researchers have reflected on working with the public on a range of projects and reported more generally on the benefits and costs. Not all the reports describe how the evidence of impact was obtained. Some articles report on a very robust process of assessing the impact of involvement, for example, gathering the views of the public and academic members of research teams via interviews, pre- and post-involvement questionnaires and focus groups. Others have taken a much simpler approach. However, the quality of the process does not always guarantee the quality of the evidence. For example, studies which have run a randomised controlled trial to assess the impact of involvement, have sometimes proved inconclusive. This is because other contextual factors have limited the significance of the results. On the other hand, some of the more 'anecdotal' accounts of involvement have provided very powerful and convincing evidence of impact. (Staley, 2009, page 24)

Approaches or models and tools of assessment

Assessing evidence can be a heavy workload. Salmon (1998) argues that 'the attempt to gain scientific understanding of the world is a complicated matter' (page 78). Depending upon the needs, there are different models and approaches of assessment or evaluation tested in different disciplines for different purposes, and these approaches provide some frameworks for assessing evidence in different contexts. As Patton (2002) notes, models often offer assessors or evaluators some structure and support. In Alkin's (1997) views, these frameworks help methodological decisions, offer guidance about the process and provide appropriate direction. Table 6.1 illustrates the taxonomy of approaches, target audiences and typical questions relevant to assessing the evidence.

Table 6.1 Taxonomy of major assessment-evaluation approaches or models

Models	*Reference groups (target audience)*	*Key relevant questions*
Public health system analysis	Health care managers, policy-planners and decision-makers	Can the public health effects be achieved more economically?
Behavioural objectives	Health care managers and practitioners	Is the programme achieving its objectives?
Decision making	Health care practitioners health care managers, health care professionals	Is the programme effective?
Goal free	Health service users/patients	What are all the intended effects?
Professional review	Health care practitioners; general public	What is the professional opinion of the programme?
Quasi-legal (adversary)	Policy-planners and decision makers; political people	What are the arguments for and against the programme?
Case study	Health service users/patients; health care practitioners	What does the programme look like to different people?

Source: Adapted from House (1978, 1986).

According to Patton (1982, 2002), some models of evaluation can be divided, based on the nature and areas of topic (Table 6.2).

Table 6.2 Models of assessment/evaluation

Models	Comments
Taylor	Evaluation by objectives
	• Outcomes criteria are based on the service users' behaviours
Scriven	Goal free
	• Needs-driven analysis – doing fieldwork and gathering data on a broad array of actual effects or outcomes, and then comparing them with the observed outcomes
	• Evaluators makes a deliberate attempt to avoid all rhetoric related to programme goals
	• The model avoids the risk of narrowly studying stated programme objectives and thereby missing important unanticipated outcomes; removes negative connotations attached to the discovery of unanticipated effects; eliminates biases and maintains assessor/evaluator independence on goals
Eisner	Connoisseurship
	• The specialist in nature that means evaluation places the evaluator's perceptions and expertise at the centre of the process
Provus	Discrepancy (ideal vs actual)
	• What people actually want to happen
	• Critical analysis of the differences
Stake	Countenance (description and judgement)
	• Focus on plans (intents) rather than outcomes (goals)
	• Description and judgement of the programme using multiple data sources and analyses
	Responsive
	• Stakeholders' involvement – be responsive to the information needs of various audiences or stakeholders; for example, assess the degree of satisfaction or dissatisfaction with the programme's effects
Stuffkebeam	CIPP (context, input, process and product)
	• Context – environment where interventions take place (e.g. socio-economic, political and cultural contexts, including institutions, target groups and peoples' interests, needs and opportunities)
	• Input – resources and capabilities
	• Process – implementation of health interventions (i.e. planning and monitoring, recording/reporting)
	• Products – outputs and outcomes (benefits)
Parlett and Hamilton	Illuminative
	• Emphasis on process and methods

Source: Adapted from Patton (1982; 2002, pages 169–180).

Types and tools of assessment/evaluation

Formulative evaluation

As discussed earlier, assessment or evaluation can be carried out for different purposes. At the beginning of any planning cycle, assessment will be performed to decide what programmes and activities or interventions to implement. Such an assessment is called a formulative nature of evaluation (Mella *et al.*, 2000, page 295). As Mella *et al.* argue, formative evaluation is designed to answer the objectives of the plan through identification of alternative health care interventions or programmes, and the selection of one of two alternatives from the set of choices. The types of assessment or evaluation that are carried out for this purpose are therefore those that assess the feasibility of public health activities or interventions in terms of 'technical effectiveness, cost effectiveness, cost-efficiency or cost-benefit analysis, political and social acceptability as well as administrative feasibility' (page 296). The decision at the end of this type of assessment would be either to adopt, or not to adopt, health care programmes or projects, or modify the health care services in the light of users' needs and interests.

Formative evaluation

This is also called process evaluation, and normally it will be carried out sometime in the middle of the programme, with the aim of assessing how the planned health care programme is progressing towards meeting the set desired purposes. In such a stage, the evaluator normally examines the evidence in the light of how the inputs (resources) are being utilised or applied. Smith *et al.* (2005, page 12) add that this approach ensures 'quality assurance and monitoring' in assessing evidence. Some relevant questions which could be asked during this stage are:

- Are the programme activities or interventions proceeding according to the plan, or are there any deviations from the original plan?

- Is the implementation of the plan on time, or is it lagging behind the set schedule?

- Are the programme activities or interventions still relevant in meeting the set desired aims?

- In terms of how the resources are set up, are they adequate to meet the desired aims?

- To what extent are other aspects of operationalisation or implementation of the health plan proceeding? (from Mella *et al.*, 2000, page 296)

The aim of the process evaluation and monitoring is to measure or assess to what extent problems or bottlenecks have emerged from the implementation, and to examine and assess them critically in order to come up with strategies to overcome these emerging issues. The lessons learned from this stage are very important for providing feedback to the top management team, particularly health policy planners and decision makers, in order for them to change or appropriately modify the 'modus operandi' of the programme implementation.

Summative evaluation

This is often the third category in assessing evidence. The key aim of the evaluation is to ascertain whether any public health programmes or health care interventions have achieved any intended objectives. Summative assessment would often attempt to measure the final results, i.e. outcomes or impacts, of the programmes. As Mella *et al.* (2000) argue, in this assessment both 'programme objectives' and 'targets' set in the planning stage are considered as principal indicators. Therefore it can be argued that best planning is always a first step to assessing any outcomes. In Mella *et al.*'s view 'evaluation is the twin sister of planning' (page 297). At this point, it may be important to distinguish between output, outcome and impact.

Input >> Output >> Outcome>> Impact

Outputs are normally considered as intermediate objectives or evidences. Some examples of outputs may be the number of health care training/education sessions, or number of children vaccinated with the BCG vaccine. Outcomes, on the other hand, are the final indicators, and may be represented by the reduction of mortality or mobility patterns of diseases or ailments, or a decrease in the mortality rate of colon cancer among patients aged 50 and over. These are usually the health status indicators that the programme intends to achieve. Impacts are considered as broader categories of outcomes in the sense that these may include the intended and unintended outcomes of any programme effects. Sometimes in order to assess impact, we have to collect information beyond health sector data; for example, to examine the impact of devolution on health services among service users, we might need to know to what extent productivity in the labour market has increased, and to what extent poverty has reduced due to a decrease in the morbidity of a certain disease. This in turn is the outcome of a disease reduction or morbidity reduction programme. Improving quality of life by improving population health and wellbeing is another good example of the impact of a health programme. A framework has been developed using these three levels of assessments (Figure 6.2).

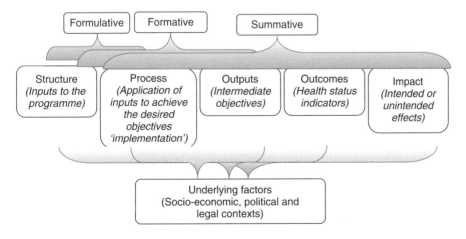

Figure 6.2 Assessment or evaluation framework.

Source: Modified and adapted from Mella *et al.* (2000, page 298).

ACTIVITY 6.4

Imagine a health care intervention with which you are familiar (a sexual health/GUM clinic for young people, or a chlamydia clinic for teenage pregnancy for example, but it could be anything at all). Specify as precisely as possible the objectives that this intervention aims to achieve, and that you would assess. Next, consider how you would measure whether the intervention actually achieves these stated objectives.

What are the key learning points that you can identify from this activity? How easy was it to apply the framework illustrated in Figure 6.2?

> Comment: In practice, there is a very limited number of tools which have been developed and tested to assess the evidence of public health outcomes (Trinder and Reynolds, 2000). Most of the tools have been used to measure competency in medical education rather than broader public health interventions (Hatala and Guyatt, 2002). Richards et al. (1995a,b) have reported that many healthcare researchers are interested in assessing public health outcomes looking from the science-based approach, and as a result there was limited scope in focusing on public topics (i.e. one level) (Mays et al., 1998), or one particular aspect of public health performance, with no emphasis on the wider 'process aspect' of measuring outcomes. Therefore Handler et al. (2001) argue that in general, a lack of conceptual framework and poor examination of impact factors, internal and external forces, are the key problems in assessing outcomes in public health systems. Handler et al. thus advocate the importance of a holistic approach encompassing 'a conceptual framework that explicates the various components of the public health (systems) and the relationships between them'.

A number of tools have been developed to assess some process aspects of evidence-based medicine and these might be applicable to public health. These include the Berlin and Fresno tools and multiple choice questionnaires, which seek to assess or measure the 'psychometric properties, objectively measured outcomes and degree of validity and reliability' (Fritsche et al., 2002; Ramos et al., 2003; Shaneyfelt et al., 2006; Iliac, 2009).

- Berlin Assessment Tool: this tool was developed by experts in evidence-based practice, with the aim of measuring the competency of medical professionals, particularly their knowledge and skills in practice, using 15 multiple choice questions (Fritsche et al., 2002). These skills and knowledge focus mostly on aspects of epidemiology, and the outcomes are compared with a control group. It can be argued that the strength of this tool (Berlin) is the ability to differentiate the expertise reliably between these two groups. However, Ilic (2009) noted that it can only assess one component of evidence, i.e. degree and level of candidates' competency in the field of epidemiology and biostatistics. Another limitation is that this tool can only assess competency in medicine, but not in other fields such as public health, nursing or allied health programmes.

- Fresno Assessment Tool: this tool also intends to measure the competency of medical professionals in evidence-based practice, particularly their knowledge and skills (Ramos *et al.*, 2003). This tool has two components – clinical scenarios with open-ended questions, and following four stages involved in the process of evidence-based practice. In terms of its strength, this tool has been validated by medical residents and has good reliability, as it has been argued that to carry out this process one requires some expert knowledge (Ilic, 2009). Ilic further claims this tool can be considered as 'standard' and is able to 'measure objectively' the participants' knowledge and skills. Miller (1990) also argues in favour of this tool as 'comprehensive', as he claims that this tool measures the wider aspects of participants' knowledge, competencies, performance and actions. Despite a wider scope of assessing competences in practice, it has limited application in medicine, as this tool can assess competency in other fields – public health, nursing or allied health programmes.

- Multiple choice questions (MCQs) and extended matching questions (EMQs): these have both been used to assess learners' competency, particularly in the area of clinical knowledge and competency (Wood, 2003).

Chapter summary

This chapter has examined the concept of evidence-based practice and ways of assessing evidence in health care interventions. It suggests that assessing or measuring evidences in any intervention is complex in nature, as patient and policy maker have different interpretations of evidence, and there are various factors that may influence planning and decision-making processes, particularly in the context of public health and health promotion, as people's health has been determined by many factors. This chapter has suggested some practical points on what to assess, and how, and most importantly where, to assess evidences using different methods and tools. This chapter has shown that although in different literatures there is an increasing trend towards using the evidence-based approach in public health, uptake to date has been limited and practical experiences are variable. The chapter concludes that assessing evidence in public health is therefore a complex task that requires both the application of a wide range of professional skills and knowledge, and the use of appropriate assessment methods and tools in practice.

Acknowledgements

The author would like to thank Dr Dragan Ilic, Monash University, Australia, for his helpful comments on an earlier draft of this chapter.

- Campbell collaboration www.campbellcollaboration.org
  The Campbell Collaboration helps people make well-informed decisions by preparing, maintaining and disseminating systematic reviews in education, crime and justice, and social welfare.

- The Cochrane Collaboration www.cochrane.org
  International not-for-profit organisation preparing, maintaining and promoting the accessibility of systematic reviews of the effects of health and health care.

- NHS Evidence www.evidence.nhs.uk/default.aspx
  NHS Evidence provides free access to clinical and non-clinical information – local, regional, national and international. Information includes evidence, guidance and Government policy.

- National Institute for Heath and Clinical Excellence www.nice.org.uk
  NICE is an organisation devoted to disseminating evidence on public health and health care effectiveness and cost-effectiveness.

chapter 7

Assessing Evidence – Cost-Effectiveness Analysis

Gary Ginsberg

Meeting the public health competences

Core area 2: Assessing the evidence of effectiveness of interventions, programmes and services to improve population health and wellbeing.

This chapter will help you to evidence the following competences for public health (Public Health Skills and Careers Framework):

- Level 6 (d) Knowledge of various techniques to assess productivity and cost-effectiveness
- Level 7 (e) Understanding of the validity and use of various techniques to assess productivity and cost-effectiveness, and the inferences that can be drawn.

This chapter will also assist you in demonstrating the following National Occupational Standard(s) for public health:

- Encourage innovation in your area of responsibility – (M&L C2)
- Facilitate the clinical audit process – (HI124)
- Develop evidence-based clinical guidelines – (HI127).

This chapter will also be useful in demonstrating Standard 7 of the Public Health Practitioner Standards.

- Standard 7. Assess the evidence of effective interventions and services to improve health and wellbeing – demonstrating:

  a. knowledge of the different types, sources and levels of evidence in own area of practice and how to access and use them
  b. the appraisal of published evidence and the identification of implications for own area of work.

Chapter overview

This chapter will help you to set priorities on the basis of evidence-based public health between various public health interventions. This chapter will help you to calculate the cost–utility ratios of public health interventions which integrate both epidemiological and economic evidence in a common rubric. Exercises in this chapter will focus on:

- estimating the savings in averted treatment costs as a result of morbidity decreases caused by the intervention;
- estimating increased quality-adjusted life years (QALYs) due to morbidity reductions caused by the intervention;
- estimating increased QALYs due to mortality reductions caused by the intervention;
- calculating the cost–utility ratio of the intervention.

Public health practitioners have to choose which of many various interventions should be adopted (and which should not be adopted or even closed). In this chapter the key epidemiologic and economic features of an intervention will be explored in order to help identify ways to decide whether to adopt or reject projects more subjectively and effectively.

Learning outcomes

After reading this chapter you will be able to:

- calculate costs and future treatment savings of interventions;
- estimate additional QALYs from morbidity and/or mortality gains from the intervention;
- prioritise projects according to their cost-effectiveness ratio (costs per QALY).

Why do we need cost-effectiveness analysis (CEA)

In the field of public health, there are numerous potential interventions, ranging from immunisations against infectious diseases (e.g. measles, HPV infections, etc.), health promotion programmes for reducing risk factors (e.g. smoking, overweight, sedentary lifestyles, etc.), screening programmes for early diagnosis of diseases (e.g. thalassaemia, colorectal cancer, etc.) as well as various treatment options (e.g. surgical, pharmaceutical, etc.). All societies (whether capitalist, socialist, communist or mixed economies) have only a limited amount of resources that they can allocate to any sector, including health, so decisions have to be made about which of the many potential public health programmes should be adopted (or not) and which existing programmes should be discontinued. Often such decisions are made through struggles between political groups, pressure groups and interest groups (professional, public, private and industrial).

A more rational, scientific, objective and evidence-based approach to prioritising programmes was made towards the end of the last century with the use of cost–benefit analysis (CBA), where expected monetary benefits and monetary costs of interventions were compared. However CBA did not directly measure (in non-monetary terms) the day-to-day health and functional (e.g. able to walk, lack of pain, etc.) benefits that individuals could receive from a successful intervention.

Cost-effectiveness analysis (CEA) basically searches for the cheapest way of achieving a given goal. CEA compares the costs of different interventions with their outcomes, often measured in terms of costs per case prevented, cost per averted death or cost per life year saved. Since the turn of the century, the major tool used for prioritisation has been a form of CEA known as cost–utility analysis (CUA), in which the outcomes are measured in terms of QALYs. Sometimes outcomes are measured in terms of costs per DALY (disability-adjusted life year).

A CUA calculates the cost per QALY (or DALY) as defined by the following formula:

$$\text{Cost per QALY} = \frac{\text{Cost of intervention} - \text{Savings from intervention}}{\text{QALYS added from decreased mortality and morbidity}}$$

How to calculate the cost–utility ratio

Stage I: Estimating costs of intervention

In measuring the costs of the intervention you are considering, you should include whatever of the following health service costs are incurred by the intervention:

- General practitioner
- Emergency room
- Day hospitalisation
- Overnight hospitalisation
- Surgery
- Laboratory tests
- Imaging
- Outpatient visits
- Rehabilitation
- Home visits
- Nursing care
- Vaccination costs (including cold-chain, transportation, monitoring, swabs, needles, serum and a provision for vaccine wastage)
- Costs of side-effects
- Other costs.

Costs (and savings) should ideally be presented from a wide societal perspective (WHO, 2006) and therefore should include not only costs falling on the health services, but also costs falling on other government bodies (e.g. education, social services) as well as costs due to:

- work absences as a result of undergoing the intervention;

- transportation costs;

- out-of pocket costs (e.g. special food).

Because of space constraints our examples will only consider costs from a health service perspective. All costs and QALYs should be subject to discounting (see Box 7.1). Project costs should be adjusted by expected coverage and compliancy rates. If these rates fall short of 100 per cent, they will reduce the intervention costs, but will also reduce the resultant health and monetary benefits of the intervention.

Example 7.1 What is discounting?

If you were offered 100 pounds today or 100 pounds one year from now, you should choose to have the money now. By having the money now, it gives you more choices (you can spend it or save it) as opposed to having no choice at all for the next year. In addition, there is a small chance (rising with age) that you will not die during the coming year and so will not benefit from (either saving or spending) the money. In order to entice us to give up the advantages of having money now, banks offer us interest to compensate ourselves for having fewer choices. Money now is therefore worth more than money in the future (even if the inflation rate is zero).

If the interest rate is 10 per cent per year, then 100 pounds invested now, will be worth

$100 \times (1 + 10\%) = 110$ pounds next year
$100 \times (1 + 10\%)^2 = 121$ pounds in two years' time
$100 \times (1 + 10\%)^3 = 133$ pounds in three years' time etc.

The general formula is that P pounds invested at $r\%$ per annum interest will be worth $P \times (1 + r\%)^n$ pounds $= F$ pounds in n years' time (a).

This process is known as compounding. The reverse process that translates money in the future (F) into its present value (P) is called discounting and utilises a formula derived from formula (a) above:

$P = F/(1 + r)^n$

For example, if interest rates are 10 per cent, then 121 pounds received two years from now is worth $121/(1 + 10\%)^2 = 100$ pounds today.

ACTIVITY 7.1

You are building a health centre in your town. If you build it with contractor A, you will have to pay 19 million pounds immediately. Contractor B will accept 10 million pounds now and 11 million next year. Contractor C will charge you 2 million pounds now, 11 million next year and a further 7.26 million two years from now. Assuming all contractors build to the same standard and interest rates are 10 per cent per annum, which contractor should you choose?

Answer

Contractor C, because the net present value (NPV) is the lowest.

- NPV of contractor A's costs is 19 million
- NPV of contractor B's costs is 20 million = 10 million + 11 million$/(1 + 10\%)^1$
- NPV of contractor C's costs is 18 million = 2 million + 11 million$/(1 + 10\%)^1$ + 7.26 million$/(1 + 10\%)^2$

A person who is unfamiliar with discounting will erroneously take on contractor A, as his or her costs total is the lowest at 19 million, compared with B or C's 21 million and 20.26 million respectively.

Stage II: Selecting a comparator

A new intervention's costs (and outcomes) should be compared with some or all of the following:

- The intervention that is currently used as standard practice (e.g. if your new intervention is the vaccination against the human papilloma virus (HPV) that causes cervical cancer, then a comparator would be PAP smears given every three years in the UK) (Ginsberg *et al.*, 2007; Goldie *et al.*, 2008).

- An alternative intervention (e.g. fecal occult blood testing vs. colonoscopy or sigmoidoscopy for discovering colorectal cancer) (Ginsberg *et al.*, 2010a).

- Doing nothing or the 'null'. This approach is recommended by the WHO, but can involve tricky calculations as to what the incidence or the case-fatality rate of a disease would be if the person received no health care at all.

In addition, the efficiency of the new intervention should be compared with the efficiency of the comparator. This will enable you to not only estimate the treatment costs averted by the intervention but also to estimate the increase in QALYs provided by the intervention.

Data on the efficiency of the intervention is usually obtained from meta-analyses (combining results) of clinical trials, which ideally should be randomised controlled trials. Paradoxically, new interventions will not have undergone many trials, especially independent trials not funded by pharmaceutical companies who have vested interests in the intervention. For diseases that are slow in progression, intermediate markers of effectiveness can be used (e.g. use the effectiveness of drugs in reducing low-density lipoprotein cholesterol levels to estimate future decreases in incidence and mortality from coronary heart disease). For diseases such as colorectal cancer, complex epidemiological models can be built to predict outcomes, since the time lag between the intervention and its effect might well run into decades.

Stage III: Estimating Future Treatment Savings

ACTIVITY 7.2

A vaccination programme against Haemophilus influenza type B (HIB) aims to vaccinate all one million children aged one who live in a region. The vaccine costs 2 pounds a dose, but 10 per cent is wasted due to having to throw away what is left open in multi-dose vials every day. Labour and other costs amount to 80 pence per dose. Each child requires three doses. Compliancy with the programme is expected to be 90 per cent. Calculate the cost of the intervention.

At present in the region there are 2000 cases of HIB annually in children aged one. For simplicity's sake we will assume that disease incidence is zero in children over two years old. Each case incurs on average 1000 pounds in health service costs (including costs of chronic sequelae). What is the annual burden of HIB in monetary terms? The vaccine has an efficacy of 95 per cent. What is the savings in averted treatment costs as a result of the vaccination? What is the net cost of the intervention?

Answer

Cost per dose is 2 pounds + 20 pence (wastage) + 80 pence plus (other costs) = 3 pounds.

Three million doses (3 doses × 1 million children) are ideally needed, but since compliance is only 90 per cent, only 2 700 000 doses will be used. Intervention cost is therefore 8 100 000 pounds.
The annual cost of HIB is 2000 × 1000 pounds = 2 000 000 pounds annually.
The vaccination programme will prevent 95% (efficacy) × 2000 cases × 90% (compliancy) = 1710 cases. Averted treatment costs are 1710 × 1000 = 1 710 000 pounds.
Net intervention costs = 8 100 000 (intervention) – 1 710 000 (averted treatment) = 6 390 000 pounds.

We can use the efficiency data to estimate the interventions impact on disease incidence, severity of disease and mortality. Reduced incidence and severity means lower utilisation of health services and hence decreased treatment costs. The cost categories listed for the costs of the intervention (Stage I) can be used as a framework to calculate the costs of the disease that the intervention is aimed at (WHO, 2009).

These averted treatment costs (appropriately discounted to take into account savings generated in future years) can be deducted from the intervention cost to give the net costs of the programme. If the averted treatment costs exceed the intervention costs (e.g. taxing tobacco or group therapy for smoking cessation; Ginsberg *et al.*, 2010b), the intervention is said to be cost-saving.

Stage IV: Estimating averted QALY losses as a result of decreased morbidity

Ideally, a person should be born completely healthy and should not suffer from one day's illness all their lifetime and then, after their 120th birthday celebration, the person should peacefully pass away in their sleep. Such a lucky person has 100 per cent health for all their 120 years. They have in effect experienced 120 times 1 (undiscounted) QALYs in their lifetime.

Unfortunately, the reality is that all of us at some time suffer from illnesses that reduce our quality of life over our lifetime. In Figure 7.1, for example, the duration of the illness is measured in terms of time (years) and appears on the horizontal axis and the vertical axis represents a health status index, where death is given the value 0 (or 0 per cent) and being totally healthy given the value 1 (or 100 per cent).

There are many different ways of creating health status indices, based on direct and indirect survey data as well as utilising questionnaires that measure the quality of life in different dimensions, such as the SF-36 (Ware, 2010) and the EuroQuol (EQ-5D, 2010). These estimate the severity of the illness but have to be multiplied by the duration of the illness in order to measure the QALY loss due to morbidity. For example, if a broken finger has a QALY weight of 0.95 (or 95 per cent, also referred to as a disability weight of $1-0.95 = 0.05$ or 5 per cent) and the disability lasts for two months, the QALY loss will be 0.05×2 months$/12$ months $= 0.00833$ QALYs.

Figure 7.1 shows the quality of life with and without an intervention for a disease (e.g. cancer) in a 60-year-old woman. The dashed line shows that if an intervention is carried out (e.g. hysterectomy and/or chemotherapy and/or radiotherapy for stage I cervical cancer) the woman's quality of life is higher than in a no-intervention scenario (unbroken line). Note that due to the natural ageing process, the quality of life gradually declines over the years. When she is 84 years old the woman contracts a fatal illness and dies.

If the woman in this example had not received the intervention, there would have been a sharp decline in their quality of life (due to fear, worry, disability, pain, etc.) and they would have died six years later, aged 66.

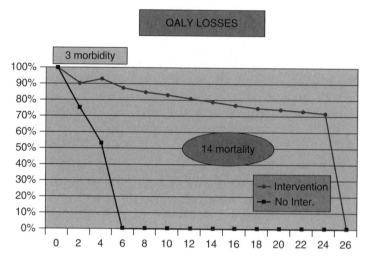

Figure 7.1 Quality-adjusted life years (QALY) losses.

The area between the two lines (and the vertical line on the horizontal axis) shows the gain in morbidity-related quality of life in the first six years due to the intervention. In our example this gain is approximately 3 (undiscounted) QALYs.

Some diseases have associated chronic sequels (e.g. deafness as a result of meningitis), which results in the person experiencing a disability for the remainder of their lifetime. The magnitude of these QALY losses is far higher than those from short-term acute morbidity, whose effects only occur over a range from a few days to a few weeks.

Stage V: Estimating averted QALY losses as a result of decreased mortality

The efficacy data from the clinical trials can be used not only to estimate the QALY loss due to morbidity but also the QALY loss due to mortality, after adjustments have been made for the natural decline in quality of life due to the ageing process. The burden of disease is the sum of the QALY losses from morbidity and mortality.

While life expectancy at birth in a developed country might be 80 years, the healthy adjusted life expectancy (HALE) might be around 68 years, because 12 QALYS have been lost (WHO, 2002) due to disabilities caused by illnesses (e.g. measles, dementia, etc.) and the natural ageing process.

Figure 7.1 shows the QALY gains of the intervention because the person does not die from the cancer six years after the intervention, but is cured and remains alive for a further 20 years. The summation of the area between the two curves shows that approximately 14 (undiscounted) QALYs will be added as a result of the intervention.

ACTIVITY 7.3

HIB cases have an associated QALY loss of 0.1 for one month. There are 2000 cases per year with a 1 per cent case fatality rate (i.e. 20 persons). A further 1 per cent of cases suffer from long-term neurological damage that result in a (discounted) QALY loss of 15 QALYs per person. Average life expectancy at age 1 is 79 years and average healthy adjusted life expectancy is 70 years.

- Calculate the burden of disease from HIB in the region.
- The vaccine has an efficiency of 95 per cent and compliancy with the programme is 90 per cent. How many undiscounted QALY losses are prevented by the vaccine?

Answer

Acute morbidity QALY loss is 2000 (cases) × 0.1 × 1 month/12 months = 2000 × 0.0165 = 33 QALYs. QALY loss due to long-term sequelae is 20 cases × 0.15 QALYS = 300 QALYs. Mortality QALY losses are 20 persons × 70 years (HALE) = 1400 QALYs. The burden of disease is 33 + 300 + 1400 = 1733 QALYs. Vaccination will prevent a 1733 × 90% (compliancy) × 95% (efficiency) = 1482 QALY loss.

Stage VI: Applying the cost per QALY formula

Here we just plug into the following formula, the components we have calculated in the previous stages:

$$\text{Cost per QALY} = \frac{\text{Cost of intervention} - \text{Savings from intervention}}{\text{QALYS added from decreased mortality and morbidity}}$$

Using standardised methodology, one can perform CUA on various new interventions. These interventions can then be ranked in terms of their costs per QALY. First, the interventions that are effective and cost-saving should be adopted (after taking into consideration other factors such as manpower availability etc.). Next, interventions that have a low cost per QALY should be adopted until the budget runs out. Adoption of a project with a high cost per QALY instead of an alternative with a low cost per QALY would effectively mean that there will be a lower decrease in morbidity and/or mortality in the population. Such a decision would have to be justified on other grounds (e.g. equity, preference for certain disease group, etc.).

ACTIVITY 7.4

From the previous activities, we have shown that the vaccination intervention will cost 8 100 000 pounds, but will save 1 710 000 pounds in averted treatment costs (Activity 7.2). The effects of the vaccination will reduce the QALY loss from acute morbidity, chronic sequelae and mortality by 1482 QALYS (Activity 7.3). Calculate the cost per QALY of the intervention. Would you recommend the adoption of the vaccination in the region?

Answer

Cost per QALY = (8 100 000 – 1 710 000)/1482 = 4312 pounds per QALY
On the basis of CUA the intervention is very cost effective.

Some countries have adopted a fixed threshold figure (say $50 000 or 30 000 pounds) below which an intervention is deemed to be cost-effective. However, a better threshold may be defined in relation to the resources available in a country as measured by gross domestic product (GDP) per head. Thus a developing country, such as Rwanda, will have a far lower threshold (due to their lower levels of resource availability) than England or the United States. As a rule of thumb, the WHO defines a project as being very cost-effective if the cost per QALY is less than the GDP per head but is greater than zero (WHO, 2001). If the cost per QALY lies between one and three times the per capita GDP, then the project is said to be cost-effective. If QALYs are bought at a cost higher than three times the per capita GDP, then the project is not cost-effective. The World Bank uses a different criterion that describes a project as being cost-effective if the cost per QALY is less than the GDP per head.

If one is unsure of the exact value of one or more of the parameters (e.g. vaccine price ranging from one to three pounds per dose), then one can carry out a sensitivity analysis over the feasible range of the parameter(s). This will generate a range of cost per QALYs which can be incorporated into the decision-making process.

Case study 7.1: Should Albania adopt a nationwide vaccination against Haemophilus influenza? (Ginsberg, 2003)

The Global Alliance for Vaccines and Immunization (GAVI) offered to fund (for five years) HIB vaccinations to countries that have a low gross national product (GNP) per capita. In 2003, the public health authorities in Albania were wary of applying for funding for two reasons:

- They did not want to take free funds for a project that might not be really needed in their country, thereby depriving another developing country the use of the funds.
- They did not want to commit to funding the project from their limited resources, after the five-year GAVI funding period.

Therefore they commissioned a quick cost–utility analysis that took five days to collect data and another two weeks to analyse.

Examination of case-notes in the major hospitals where children with meningitis and pneumonia caused by HIB were treated, enabled the calculation of incidence and mortality rates in addition to estimates to be made of the costs of treatment. Because of the limited time period of the study, data on QALY losses from meningitis and pneumonia as well as QALY losses, incidence rates and costs of (subsequently adjusted to Albanian cost levels) were obtained from internationally published literature.

Based on a 95 per cent vaccine efficacy rate (from clinical trials) and a 98 per cent national coverage rate (the same as Albania's coverage rate for diphtheria vaccinations), it was calculated that vaccination will reduce the annual incidence of HIB meningitis and pneumonia from 35 to 2.5 cases and from 175 to 13 cases respectively. Deaths will fall from 4.5 to 0.4 cases for meningitis and 26 cases to 2.7 cases for pneumonia. These estimates can be considered to be conservative as the calculation did not take into account the more complex issue of the generation of herd immunity (to unvaccinated children) by the programme.

Life expectancy at age one was 74 years, with a HALE of 62.3 years. The vaccination programme would prevent the loss of 1835 QALYs (93 per cent from mortality, 7 per cent from morbidity). The total cost of the intervention was US$844 000 or US$16.35 per child, of which vaccine costs (including wastage) accounted for 57 per cent, labour 36 per cent, clinic overheads 3.5 per cent and surveillance, transport, side-effects, cold-chain and injection safety boxes for needle disposal the remaining 3.5 per cent. Costs per case were US$502 for meningitis and US$300 for pneumonia.

The vaccination will save US$40 000 in averted acute care costs, but this is exceeded by a (discounted) savings of US$54 000 in averted care costs for chronic sequelae, due to the long-term provision of institutional care, sheltered workshops and special education. Therefore the net costs of the intervention to the health services was US$844 000 – 40 000 – 54 000 = US$750 000, giving a cost per QALY of US$409 from a health services perspective.

In addition there was a saving of US$2000 in parents' work losses to look after sick children and US$112 000 in lost productivity of persons suffering from long-term sequelae. So the net costs from a societal perspective of the intervention was US$636 000 (750 000 − 2000 − 112 000) or US$347 per QALY.

A sensitivity analysis that assumed the vaccine efficacy would only be 80 per cent (since real life efficacy is often lower than under trial conditions), increased the cost per QALY to US$430.

The conclusion was the vaccination should be adopted as the cost per QALY (even under the low effectiveness assumption) is considerably lower than Albania's GNP of US$1120 per capita. The vaccine will be a good use of GAVI resources for the next five years and can be justified to be funded by Albania after the five-year period has ended.

Chapter summary

In this chapter we were made aware of the need to prioritise between the many potential public health interventions. The numbers and scale of many public health and health promotion projects makes prioritisation extremely important. Effective prioritisation ensures that the public receives the maximum amount of health gains (as measured by QALYs) within the available resource constraints.

In order to make the prioritisation process as objective and scientific as possible, we should use the tool of cost-effectiveness analysis, of which cost–utility analysis is the current gold standard. In order to calculate the costs per QALY of an intervention we learned the following steps:

- How to calculate the costs of an intervention

- How to estimate the savings in averted treatment costs as a result of morbidity decreases caused by the intervention

- How to estimate the increased quality adjusted life years (QALYs) due to morbidity reductions caused by the intervention

- How to estimate the increased QALYs due to mortality reductions caused by the intervention

- How to calculate the cost–utility ratio.

GOING FURTHER

- WHO (2000) *Immunization Costing and Financing. A tool and users guide for comprehensive multi-year planning (cMYP)*. Geneva: WHO. http://whqlibdoc. who.int/hq/2006/WHO_IVB_06.15_eng.pdf
  An in-depth guide to costing immunisation programmes.

- Tan-Torres Edeger, T, Baltussen, R, Adam, T, Hutubessy, R, Acharya, A, Evans, DB and Murray, CJL eds (2003) *Generalized Cost-effectiveness, A Guide*. WHO Geneva. www.who.int/choice/publications/p_2003_generalised_cea. pdf
  Provides an in-depth look at the theory of generalized cost-effectiveness analysis.

- WHO (2009) *Guide to Identifying the Economic Consequences of Disease and Injury*. Geneva: WHO. www.who.int/choice/publications/d_economic_ impact_guide.pdf
  An in-depth guide to identifying the potential economic benefits of interventions to both the health services and society as a whole.

- WHO CHOICE (Choosing Interventions that are Cost effective) www.who. int/choice/en/
  This website provides cost–utility ratios for a wide variety of public health intervention for different regions in the world, based on a standardized methodology.

chapter 8

Principles and Methods of Programme Evaluation

Carmen Aceijas

Meeting the public health competences

Core area 2: Assessing the evidence of effectiveness of interventions, programmes and services to improve population health and wellbeing.

This chapter will help you to evidence the following competences for public health (Public Health Skills and Careers Framework):

- Level 7 (d) Knowledge of the principles and methods of evaluation, audit, research and development, and standard setting, as applied to improving quality.

This chapter will also assist you in demonstrating the following National Occupational Standard(s) for public health:

- Assess the evidence and impact of health and healthcare – (PHS07) interventions, programmes and services and apply the assessments to practice
- Improve the quality of health and healthcare interventions and services through audit and evaluation – (PHS08)
- Support and challenge workers on specific aspects of their practice – (CJ F309).

Chapter overview

This chapter presents principles and methods of evaluation and improvement of public health interventions and programmes. It provides a comprehensive theoretical framework for the evaluation of public health programmes.

Exercises in this chapter will focus on:

- developing clarity about the process of planning a program evaluation;
- testing skills in programme evaluation planning;
- reviewing and consolidating knowledge on programme evaluation.

As a generic term 'evaluation' is defined as 'systematic investigation of the merit, worth, or significance of an object' (Scriven, 1998). This chapter is occupied specifically with public health programme evaluation as an essential organisational practice in public health (Dyal, 1995) aiming to systematically examine programmes/ interventions to improve them. The duty to evaluate public health actions through the systematic examination of its value and the detection of room for improvement is obvious, but another reason, running in parallel to the aim of improvement, is the need to guarantee the accountability of public health actions given that they exist thanks to public funding and they always pursue the public health protection and improvement.

Learning outcomes

After reading this chapter you will be able to:

- identify the nature and main features of programme evaluation;
- understand the main concepts and mechanisms behind public health programme evaluation;
- be familiar with the process of designing and implementing a programme evaluation.

Principles of programme evaluation

Programme evaluation should be guided by the operating principles for public health activities. Such operating principles have been extensively articulated throughout the literature on evidence-based public health and programme evaluation, but in this chapter we recall the principles adopted by the Centers for Disease Control and Prevention (CDC, 1999) from the classic papers by Dyal (1995) and Koplan (1999):

- using science as a basis for decision making and public health action;

- expanding the quest for social equity through public health action;

- performing effectively as a service agency;

- making efforts outcome-oriented; and

- being accountable.

Such operating principles implicitly demand that public health activities are clearly designed, planned, managed and evaluated. For example:

- Only programmes that have been clearly planned with a thorough background of examination of existing evidence regarding effectiveness and efficacy of services targeting a given public health issue can claim that they use 'science as a basis for decision-making'.

- Only programmes submitted to continuous or routine evaluations can guarantee the principle of 'performing effectively'.

- Only programmes that operate under clear programmes can be identified as credible programmes in terms of the principle of 'making efforts outcome-orientated'.

Furthermore, programmes guided by the above listed principles will need an array of tools (e.g. feedback systems, informative partnerships, and so on) to enable the process of continuous learning and improvement.

In addition to the operating principles of any public health programme evaluation, three main considerations will apply in deciding the procedures to be applied:

- The evaluation will be feasible,

- The evaluation will both be ethical and will examine the ethical quality of the intervention, and

- Procedures and how they will combine in the evaluation exercise will result in accurate assessment of the intervention.

A framework for public health programme evaluation

In this section a generic framework for public health programme evaluation is presented. Such a framework defines the evaluation process as six generic steps that will have to be tailored for the specific programme's assessment objective and, although they are presented and described in a consecutive way, in practice they will hardly be followed in a linear sequence. In fact, findings in any of the steps 2–5 will be likely to force the evaluating team to reconsider previous steps. However, the design of an evaluation exercise around well-structured steps will permit the evaluation to be a systematic and consistent exercise granted with the necessary credibility and likely to produce findings that will improve the programme to be evaluated.

The six steps for evaluation of public health programmes are (CDC, 1999):

- Step 1: Engage stakeholders

- Step 2: Describe the programme

- Step 3: Focus the evaluation design

- Step 4: Gather credible evidence

- Step 5: Justify conclusions

- Step 6: Ensure use and share lessons learned.

Step 1: Engage stakeholders

The credibility of an evaluation will be largely compromised or guaranteed and reinforced by the perceptions of stakeholders regarding the robustness of such evaluation.

Public health programmes are designed and implemented in partnerships, often involving the cooperation of different organisations, and are the product of value systems owned by the different partners. No evaluation can succeed without a clear understanding of the existing underlying value systems, operating practices and perspectives from the different partners, and the evaluation findings are likely to be criticised or dismissed should the partners consider that their own perspectives were misunderstood or not taken into account. Furthermore, the engagement of partners will guarantee that the following steps of the evaluation will be facilitated; if the stakeholders consider that the evaluation is part of 'what they do', they will tend to actively contribute in the evaluation. Hence, this first step should be approached with extreme professionalism and care, and the first task will involve the identification of stakeholders or groups of stakeholders.

In general, stakeholders are those having an investment in what will be learned and what will be done with the knowledge generated by the evaluation. They can be individuals or organisations. A traditional classification of groups of stakeholders identifies them as (CDC, 1999):

- those involved in programme operations;
- those served or affected by the programme; and
- primary users of the evaluation.

Those involved in programme operations form an eclectic group of professionals with knowledge and involvement at the operational level of the programme. Among them we can identify sponsors, collaborators, coalition partners, funding officials, administrators, managers and staff. Because of their close involvement in the programme they have valuable knowledge on how the programme is run and the potential deviations from the design of the programme. Programmes do change over time and it is not always easy to identify such changes from formal/written sources of information. Therefore their contribution is crucial for successful evaluation. However, and precisely because of their close involvement in the programme, they could perceive the evaluation as a judgement exercise on their professional practice. It is therefore very important to clearly define the boundaries between the evaluation team and stakeholders at the programme operational levels.

Those served or affected by the programme will be persons or organisations affected directly or indirectly by the programme. Among direct and indirect beneficiaries we can identify clients, family members, neighbourhood organisations, academic institutions, elected officials, advocacy groups, professional associations, sceptics, opponents, and staff of related or competing organisations. Direct beneficiaries of a programme include those who receive its services (e.g. youngsters receiving the services of a HIV prevention programme; information and means on how to prevent HIV infection), while indirect beneficiaries are typically those who benefit from the outcomes of the programme (e.g. communities where HIV infection rates are reduced or reversed thanks to the impact of the HIV prevention programme). Both direct and indirect recipients of the programme activities and impact should be involved in the evaluation and their input is especially important in the gathering of information about users' perceptions and programme impact. Antagonism to the programme agents should also be considered and attention to the root cause of the opposition (e.g. opposition to the HIV prevention programme coming from opposition to the use of condoms; opposition not to the programme but to the use of the facilities that the programme uses for its given activities). The inclusion of the views of those not supporting the programme will increase the credibility of the evaluation.

As for primary users of the evaluation, these are people in a position to take action regarding the programme or, in other words, a subset of stakeholders with management capacity in the programme evaluated. The identification of such a group should occur at the very beginning and the evaluation and their engagement should be pursued through continuous interaction with them and a commitment to include their unique information needs in the evaluation.

ACTIVITY 8.1

Can you reflect on the relative importance of the three primary types of programme stakeholders?

Step 2: Describe the programme

During this stage obtaining a clear picture of the programme characteristics, aims and strategies should be the focus of those engaged in its evaluation. Questions to be asked include those such as 'What is the programme's capacity to effect change?', 'How well developed is the programme in reference to the intended extent?', 'How does this programme fit into its context?' (community, organisation hosting it, other surrounding programmes). This is the step where the underlying theories and hypothesis (whether articulated or not during the programme design phase when the programme was conceived) can emerge more clearly. It can assist in connecting the programme components to its intended effects. Different models to test the theories behind public health programmes have been expressed, from the simple and classic experimental trial where a given programme is analysed as a treatment and the hypothesis tested is about whether the treatment provides the intended outcome, to the 'theories of change' and 'realist theories' that represent models to uncover and analyse the internal processes in a given programme (Figure 8.1).

In any case, a clear description will produce multiple advantages for the evaluation and increase its chances of success. For example:

- Since stakeholders might have differing ideas regarding the programme goals and purposes, a description of the programme that succeeds in capturing a consensual view of the programme's object of evaluation (its tools and aims) will enhance the engagement of stakeholders and the evaluation's credibility.

- A programme description that includes its processes and spells out inputs and outputs will help to focus the evaluation design.

- Such a description will also facilitate the evidence gathering by providing a clear identification of the programme components from where data will be extracted.

- It will justify the conclusions as they will be linked to the descriptive exercise of the programme. Furthermore, a correct description will enable comparisons with other similar programmes.

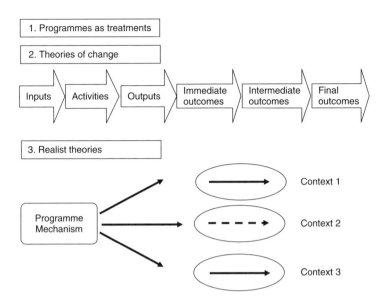

Figure 8.1 Formalising programme theories.

Source: Pawson and Sridharan (2010, page 49).

Aspects to include in a programme description are: need, expected effects, activities, resources, stage of development, context, and logic model. The need for the programme is the description of the problem(s) the programme aims to correct. The operationalisation of such problem(s) should include as much specificity as possible. For example, the magnitude of the problem, the populations affected and dynamic aspects/observed trends of the problem.

The description of expected effects equals the definition of the aspirations of a programme, its aims and objectives and it will automatically define the core indicators for measuring the success of the programme. Such description must be bounded to both the general and specific aspirations of the programme (general aims and specific objectives, immediate and long-term effects and so on) and framed in the timescale considered during the implementation of the programme. Additional attention should be paid to the unintended effects of the programme.

Responding to the question 'What does the programme do to cause the intended effects?' is equivalent to the description of its activities. They should be described as per their logical sequence, allowing the emergence of relationships between activities (how a given activity leads to the next one) and providing tests of the hypothesis and/or theories of change in the programme foundations.

The description of the resources used or at the disposal of a programme should be described as linked to the activities uncovered ('What is used for what?'). Resources include not only financial assets but also time, technology, equipment, information, human capital and so on. In addition, the economic evaluation of a programme will require the description of direct and indirect inputs and costs.

The stage of development of a programme defines what should be expected as satisfactory outcomes of an evaluation. Three main stages in the development of a programme (its level of maturity) are usually described: planning, implementation and effects, and at each stage the goal of an evaluation will be different. Thus, during the planning phase, the evaluation goal will be to refine plans, at the implementation stage (when the programme activities are field-tested) the evaluation will aim to characterise its activities in real life (as opposed to the characterisation that would take place at planning stage) and, finally, at the effects stage the programme is expected to be mature enough to have produced the intended effects. It will be time, therefore, for the evaluation to focus on the pure accountability of the programme –'Does it do what it was meant to?' – without neglecting the analysis of unintended effects as well (CDC, 1999).

The description of settings and contextual influences is the context description that includes history, geography, social and economic conditions and so on will allow a context-sensitive evaluation.

Finally, the logic model description will feed and emerge from the descriptions above but it will mark the culmination of the programme description. In a nutshell, the logic model of a programme is 'a depiction of a programme showing what the programme will do and what it is to accomplish, a series of "if–then" relationships that, if implemented as intended, lead to the desired outcomes and the core of programme planning and evaluation' (Taylor-Powell and Henert, 2008, page 55). It usually takes the shape of a graphical representation of inputs, outputs and outcomes of a programme and although many other synonyms have been used to describe it – theory of change, programme action, model of change, conceptual map, outcome map, programme logic and so on – they are all names for the process by which a programme's main structural and dynamic characteristics are displayed in relation to its intended and unintended impact. An example of the logic model, describing a programme aiming to improve water quality by reducing the concentration of diet-related phosphorus for cattle is presented in Figure 8.2.

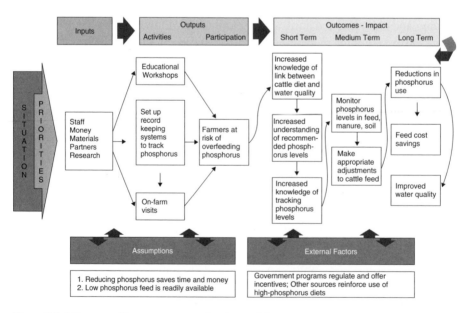

Figure 8.2 Water quality programme. Logic model.

Source: Taylor-Powell and Henert handouts (2008, page 23).

ACTIVITY 8.2

Thinking about a public health intervention that you are familiar with can you identify each of these elements and how they might be used to develop a programme
description.

ACTIVITY 8.3

After reading the case study below and using the logic model template provided
afterwards (Figure 8.3) try to fill it in with required elements. Some have been
already included to facilitate your task. Note that medium- and long-term effects
of the programme are not reported here. What do you think those effects might be?
(describe them in the chart).

Case study 8.1

Food-borne diseases remain an important cause of morbidity in the
United States among all age groups. A potentially important contribu-
tor to this morbidity is improper food handling and preparation practices in kitchens. In 2006, Los Angeles County Department of Public
Health (LACDPH) launched the Home Kitchen Self-Inspection Program, a voluntary self-inspection and education programme, to promote safer food hygiene practices at home.

The Home Kitchen Self-Inspection Program includes a Food Safety
Quiz that is based on emerging evidence that the use of online,
interactive learning tools are conducive to problem-based learning,
improve self-efficacy and self-mastery of selected skills, and offer
convenience and flexibility to the learner. The content of the questions was guided by food safety education principles from the US
Department of Agriculture: clean, separate, cook and chill. The framework of the quiz was based on adult learning theories and emphasised
such food-handling practices as the need to clean and sanitise cut-
ting boards after handling poultry, the safe handling of raw eggs, and
appropriate methods for the refrigeration of cooked and uncooked
foods.

The quiz queried respondents regarding food handling and preparation practices at home, assigning a letter grade at completion using a
scoring algorithm (i.e. A: 90–100 per cent, B: 80–89 per cent, C: 70–79
per cent). The quiz provided valuable instruction to respondents about

better ways to maintain home food safety. Respondents who received an A rating were mailed a placard with this grade as recognition for their good food-handling practices.

During the first three months after launch, the quiz was marketed to the public using printed materials and public service announcements in the local media, including television and radio, and at public events.

Approximately 13 000 adults completed the quiz; 34 per cent received an A rating, 27 per cent a B, 25 per cent a C, and 14 per cent received a numeric score because they scored lower than 70 per cent on the self-assessment. Use of interactive, online learning tools such as the Food Safety Quiz can be used to promote home food safety in the community.

Source: Adapted from CDC (2010)

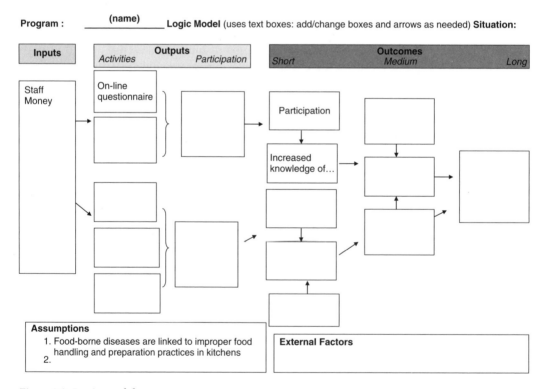

Figure 8.3 Logic model.

Source: Adapted from Taylor-Powell and Henert (2008, page 30).

Step 3: Focus the evaluation design

An evaluation of a programme involves a prioritised decision process. Not all the potential aspects of a given programme will be included in an evaluation but only those that are of the greatest concerns for stakeholders. Such decisions will suggest what design the evaluation will adopt. Once the design of the evaluation is decided, the flexibility (in terms of including other aspects not considered a priori, looking at operational issues from a different angle and so on) will be dramatically reduced. It is therefore important that the design, the plan or strategy for the evaluation, is thorough and able to anticipate the intended uses. The main points to consider when focusing an evaluation will be: purpose, users, uses, question, methods and agreements (CDC, 1999).

Public health programme evaluations have four main purposes (CDC, 1999):

- to gain insight;
- to change practice;
- to assess effects (on the programme); and
- to affect participants.

Purposes are intimately related to the uses that the evaluation will have. The recipients of the evaluation findings will be the users – individuals who utilise, in one way or other, the findings of the evaluation for the improvement of the programme. As for the questions to be answered through the evaluation, they refer to the aspects of the programme that must be investigated. The articulation of such questions will establish the boundaries of the evaluation (which aspects of the programme are tested). The methods an evaluation plan will use are usually drawn from scientific research options. The main umbrella classification for scientific designs – experimental, quasi-experimental and observational (Sim and Wright, 2000) – will be used to produce the specific design of each evaluation, taking into account the nature of the questions that are proposed. Such choices will also inform what data collection methods are available. In any case, the decision of what design to use should be driven by the need to identify the best option available to answer the evaluation questions. All designs have advantages, biases and limitations and in programme evaluation a mixed-method approach is the one that generally produces a more effective design. Finally, agreements are necessary to spell out (with minimum potential for future disagreement) the roles and responsibilities of those involved in the evaluation but they also include statements regarding the use of resources, (e.g. how the evaluation budget will be used), how ethical questions will be resolved (e.g. how to guarantee the confidentiality of users' testimonials regarding the value of the service provided by the programme).

Step 4: Gather evidence

Whether the questions posed to the programme are answered in a comprehensive and systematic way that provides the evaluation findings with sufficient credibility is largely enabled by the type of data gathered and what such data allows the evaluation team do. Depending on the design, or rather, the type of mixed-method design defined in the previous phase, the evaluation will be fed by different data collection methods, and the nature of the data itself will also be different. Thus, while some questions might require the standards of a controlled experiment, others might require the systematic observation of interactions, examination of written records and so on. In any case the selection of indicators and the sources of information are of specific relevance here. An overview of the methods for data collection widely used in programme evaluation is presented in Table 8.1. Other aspects that concern the process of gathering evidence include issues around the quality and quantity of data and sources used and the logistics required for the data collection process itself.

ACTIVITY 8.4

Can you name one advantage and one disadvantage of each of the suggested methods of data collection for programme evaluation?

The choice of indicators to be used is, once again, a matter for the questions regarding the programme that are the focus of the evaluation. They provide the basis for the definition of what evidence should be gathered. There are a multitude of indicators typically used for programme evaluation. Some of them are indicators of programme activities such as the programme's delivery of services, participation rate, client satisfaction, efficiency of resources used and so on, while others are measures of programme effects, such as changes in participant behaviour, health status, quality of life and so on. Risks in defining the indicators to be measured include the inclusion of too many indicators that might move the evaluation 'out of focus' or the indicators that are not directly related to the programme's activities that expect direct outcomes. The logical model developed in the previous step should help to identify the spectrum of indicators required – those that can be measured by the different activities of the programme. An added advantage to this system of defining indicators is that small changes, attributable to specific activities of the programme, will be visible faster. In contrast, assessing a programme with only global indicators of performance will only detect major changes, leading to potentially disappointing and misleading findings regarding the ability of the programme to honour its aims.

Step 5: Justify conclusions

The conclusions of an evaluation will be justified against the evidence obtained, and according to the standards set up a priori against the agreements taken with stakeholders. Standards defined a priori are the set of values with which stakeholders

Table 8.1 Overview of methods of collecting information

Method	Aim	Advantages	Disadvantages
Questionnaires, surveys, checklists	To collect relevant number of impersonal data quickly	Anonymous data Large quantities of data Inexpensive administration Easy comparison and analysis Large numbers of respondents Already validated and simple questionnaires available	Multiple potential sources of bias (from wording, to sample selection and including administration methods) Felt as impersonal If surveys: need of experts in the technique (e.g.: for sampling) Doesn't get full story
Interviews	To fully understand the issue investigated from the actors' perspective	In-depth information Develops relationship with client Can be flexible with client	Time-consuming Difficult analysis Prevents generalisation Costly Multiple sources of bias (e.g. interviewer's bias)
Documentation review (e.g. applications, finances, memos, minutes, etc.)	To obtain information on how the program operates without interrupting it.	Comprehensive, factual and historical information No disruption of programme's activities Doesn't require new data collection Few potential biases	Time-consuming Available data might lack of sufficient quality or completeness Restricted to existing data
Observation	To gather accurate information on operational aspects of a programme	Testimonial information on programme's process as they occur Highly adaptable to events as they evolve	Interpretation of live behaviours is difficult Categorisation of observations is complex Observation can influence behaviours of participants Costly
Focus groups	To explore a topic in depth through group discussion	Provides quickly and reliably common impressions Efficient way to get much in-depth information	Difficult analysis Need a well-trained facilitator Difficult to schedule (6–8 people together)
Case studies	To fully depict client's experiences in a programme, and conduct comprehensive examination through cross-comparison of cases	Fully description of client's experience Powerful means to portray programme to outsiders	Time-consuming Represents depth of information, rather than breadth

Source: Adapted from McNamara (2000).

believe the programme is aligned. Analytic activities applied to the data collected (data analysis) must allow the evaluation team the deconstruction achievements and milestones at the programme activities' level and must allow to the emergence of the global picture regarding the impact of the programme.

Some of the evaluation activities that will help to justify its conclusions are as follows (Joint Committee on Standards for Educational Evaluation, 1994):

- using appropriate methods of analysis and synthesis to summarise findings;

- interpreting the significance of results for deciding what the findings mean;

- making judgements according to clearly stated values that classify a result (e.g. as positive or negative and high or low);

- considering alternative ways to compare results (e.g. compared with programme objectives, a comparison group, national norms, past performance or needs);

- generating alternative explanations for findings and indicating why these explanations should or should not be discounted;

- recommending actions or decisions that are consistent with the conclusions; and

- limiting conclusions to situations, time periods, persons, contexts and purposes for which the findings are applicable.

Step 6: Ensure use and share lessons learned

The translation of evaluation findings and the recommendations generated into decision-making processes leading to actions is not automatic, nor can it be assumed by the evaluation team as something alien to the evaluation itself. Rather, it requires careful planning that will start at the beginning of the process with the engagement of stakeholders. How will this evaluation inform your practice? is a question for the evaluation team to propose to stakeholders and the answer must be a joint effort of these, at least, two parties. If the design of the evaluation was clear to the professionals involved in the programme and the different parts of the design (especially the breakdowns of evaluations per activity sets) communicated as future sources of information for the practice improvement, the evaluation would be half way to success in its purpose of becoming a useful tool for improvement. However, other issues deserve further considerations too. Thus, careful preparation for communicating the findings must be made, especially the communication of negative findings. Potential hostile reactions from programme participants or users who might feel their performance questioned must be managed so as to fully transmit the idea that the evaluation is (potentially) a credible source for improvement.

For such a purpose, the communication of findings must explain from what specific sources of evidence a given finding emerges and what suggestions for improvement are at hand. The feedback on the evaluation is not only a right of the programme participants but an opportunity for improvement of the evaluation itself by, for instance, correcting information or adding new information that somehow was missed. Finally, technical and emotional support should be provided for the follow-up of the evaluation and to prevent the lessons learnt not being fully utilised for the improvement of the programme.

Chapter summary

This chapter opens with the definition of public health programme evaluation as an essential organisational practice in public health (Dyal, 1995) aiming to systematically examine programmes/interventions to improve them.

The operating principles of programmes evaluations (a) using science as a basis for decision making and public health action; (b) expanding the quest for social equity through public health action; (c) performing effectively as a service agency; (d) making efforts outcome oriented; and (e) being accountable – were introduced. We also discussed the main considerations of programme evaluation: the evaluation will be feasible, the evaluation will both be ethical and will examine the ethical quality of the intervention, and procedures and how they will combine in the evaluation exercise will result in accurate assessment of the intervention.

The introductory contents of this chapter provided the right setting to approach the framework for public health programme evaluations which occupied the main body of this chapter. A framework structured the main steps of a programme evaluation as:

- Step 1: Engage stakeholders
- Step 2: Describe the programme
- Step 3: Focus the evaluation design
- Step 4: Gather evidence
- Step 5: Justify conclusions
- Step 6: Ensure use and share lessons learned.

Throughout the chapter you were made aware of the main activities and points for consideration at every step; from the definition of stakeholders, to the outline of the evaluation design and the main available data collection methods and including the development of the logic model and set of indicators to be used. The latest steps of the framework include considerations on communication of the findings and follow-up activities.

- Program Development and Evaluation Unit, University Of Wisconsin-Extension www.uwex.edu/ces/pdande/index.html
  The Program Development and Evaluation Unit provides training and technical assistance that enables Cooperative Extension campus and community-based faculty and staff to plan, implement and evaluate high-quality educational programmes. Their website contains a multitude of didactic materials focusing on programme evaluation. It is one of the sources routinely used by organisations like CDC and WHO for their work in programme evaluation in the health sectors.

- World Health Organisation. Monitoring and Evaluation Systems Strengthening Tool (MESST) www.theglobalfund.org/documents/me/M_E_Systems_Strengthening_Tool.pdf
  MESST is a tool designed under the auspices of several UN agencies and programmes – WHO, the Global Fund to fight HIV, Tuberculosis and Malaria, USAID and so on – to assess monitoring and evaluation (M&E) plans and systems by assessing data collection, reporting, and management systems to measure indicators of the success of programmes and projects. It addresses the M&E plan and systems that need to be in place to collect and channel data up a system for aggregation into relevant indicators for programme management and reporting. Among other advantages, MESST can be used at the national level, within groups of projects, and within individual projects or organisations.

- Salabarría-Peña, Y, Apt, BS and Walsh, CM (2007) Practical Use of Program Evaluation among sexually transmitted disease (STD) programs. Atlanta, GA: Centers for Disease Control and Prevention (CDC). Department of Health and Human Services. www.cdc.gov/std/program/pupestd.htm
  This document provides an example of practical, step-by-step applications of the framework for programme evaluation introduced in this chapter and is therefore of unquestionable use for readers willing to see a practical demonstration of how the framework with its six steps works in real public health programme evaluation.

chapter 9

Assessing Quality and Effectiveness to Improve Public Health and Wellbeing

Carmen Aceijas and Krishna Regmi

Meeting the public health competences

Core area 2: Assessing the evidence of effectiveness of interventions, programmes and services to improve population health and wellbeing.

This chapter will help you to evidence the following competences for public health (Public Health Skills and Careers Framework):

- Level 8 (a) Understanding of the principles and methods of evaluation, audit, research and development, and standard setting, as applied to improving quality.

This chapter will also assist you in demonstrating the following National Occupational Standard(s) for public health:

- Assess the evidence and impact of health and healthcare – (PHS07) interventions, programmes and services and apply the assessments to practice
- Improve the quality of health and healthcare interventions and services through audit and evaluation – (PHS08).

Chapter overview

Quality has recently been given more concern in health care than before, but the word 'quality' has several different meanings in different contexts as the facet of quality is multidimensional. For example, in the physical and medical sciences, quality is mostly concerned with the aspect of systems, whereas in social science, quality is considered with the people and their expectations, in particular the aspect of care and intervention. In this chapter, we explore the understanding of quality, purpose and significance that underpins efforts to promote public health by making health care interventions effective.

Learning objectives

After completing the chapter you will be able to:

- critically understand the concept of quality and its role in public health and health care;

- discuss some tools and measures of quality and effectiveness;
- reflect on the relationships between quality and effectiveness;
- understand the role of audit as a quality improvement tool.

Introduction

Come, give us a taste of your quality

(William Shakespeare, Hamlet, Act II, Scene ii)

From the time of Hippocrates to date, the quest for quality has always been there. Rillon (2000, page 290), however, argued that quality has been intensified with the increased attention, not only from health care, but also from the following:

- Service user pressure groups in many countries – currently the recipients are more aware of their health and their rights in terms of what they are supposed to get from health care services or service providers.

- Sky-rocketing costs demand greater efficiency – health care services have become more expensive, with the result that both users and providers are now more conscious of getting their money's worth.

- Third-party payers – health care services today have also become more complicated with the entrance of third-party payers, for example, insurance agents, and health management organisations are demanding accountability and responsibility regarding benefits to costs.

- New technology – the industrial age has also created new technology, competition and changes in best practice.

Quality in health care is complex and multidimensional in nature, but its role has been well recognised in health care and it can be defined as its dimensions of quality in health services (Maxwell, 1992, page 171):

1. Accessibility: can patients get the health care services where and when they need them?

2. Equity: do all patients with the same need get the same care? Are they fairly treated?

3. Acceptability: are these health care services provided in a way that is acceptable and that promotes patient satisfaction?

4. Effectiveness: does the health care intervention or treatment produce the intended effects?

5. Efficiency: is the care provided at reasonable cost, with little waste?

6. Relevance: are the services in accordance with the needs of the population?

ACTIVITY 9.1

Reflection: What are some strengths and weakness of each dimension of quality in health care? How would these principles translate into public health programmes? Discuss your points with your neighbour or a colleague and make any necessary changes after discussion.

A specific definition of quality in the context of public health has been produced by the US Public Health Quality Forum. They define quality in public health as: 'The degree to which policies, services, and research for the population increases desired health outcomes and conditions in which the population can be healthy' (US Department of Health and Human Services, 2008, page 3). The same group (page 5) stated that to be acknowledged as quality practices, public health interventions should be:

- Population-centred: The protection of the health of the whole population is crucial to public health interventions.

- Equitable: Public health interventions must aim to achieve health equity.

- Proactive: Public health must act timely and be able to mobilise resources rapidly to address emergencies or vulnerabilities as soon as they are detected.

- Health promoting: Health providers must operate with safe practice and public health interventions must be those that increase the probability of positive health behaviours and outcomes.

- Risk-reducing: Public health works for the diminishing of harmful environmental and social events. Its tools include the implementation of policies and strategies to reduce the odds of preventable injuries and illnesses.

- Vigilant: Public health mandate includes the surveillance of the health of the population and therefore must intensify practices and policies that support the monitoring of the health of the populations.

- Transparent: Public health practices must be open to accountability and will make valid, reliable, timely and meaningful data, available to stakeholders.

- Effective: Public health must justify investments in health care by utilising evidence regarding best practices to achieve its goals.

- Efficient: Cost and benefits of public health interventions must be clear and aimed at an optimal use of resources.

In the UK, the main document on quality in health services is still the 'High Quality Care for All. NHS Next Stage Review Final Report', which presented the findings of the initiative led by Lord Darzi. This spelled out the challenges for quality improvement within NHS and cited the following aims (Department of Health–NHS, 2008, page 33):

- Help people to stay healthy by working more effectively with national and local partners that focus on promoting health and ensuring easier access to prevention services.

- Empower patients by giving them more rights and control over their own health and personal care within the NHS.

- Provide the most effective treatments by an improved access to treatment and by promotion of early diagnosis systems.

- Keep patients as safe as possible by striving to make the NHS the safest health system, keeping patients in clean environments where avoidable harm is reduced.

The review concluded that quality in the NHS should focus on three main aspects (Department of Health–NHS, 2008, page 47):

- Patient safety – aims to secure that no harm is done to patients. It translates into efforts to secure that the health care environment is safe and clean and avoidable harm is reduced by, for instance, reducing excessive drug errors and health care-associated infection rates.

- Patient experience – this addresses the need to provide personalised care and issues such as compassion, dignity and respect towards the patient are included. The review acknowledges that only improved analysis of patient satisfaction can provide the necessary knowledge for quality improvement in this area.

- Effectiveness of care – this involves the correct understanding of success rates by analysis of measures such as mortality or survival rates, complication rates and measures of clinical improvement. An innovation of this review was the inclusion of patient-reported outcomes measures (PROMs), which include for the first time, the patients' perspective on how effective the treatment received was.

These aspects became the three dimensions for quality improvement strategies and indicators used by the NHS. In addition, the review envisaged seven steps to quality improvement (Department of Health–NHS, 2008, page 48):

- Bring clarity to quality – with the subsequent definition of high-quality care by specialty to be used to set up standards.

- Measure quality – this ensures that improvement of services can be worked out and measured. For this purposes, the review advocates a quality measurement framework at every level.

- Publish quality performance – making data available to stakeholders (staff, patients and the public) will allow understanding of the variations and best practices found in the quest for improvement.

- Recognise and reward quality – by engineering the right incentives to support quality improvement.

- Raise standards – by empowering patients and professionals. The review also defends a stronger role for clinical leadership and management throughout the NHS.

- Safeguard quality – by the clear regulation of professions and services that reassure patients and the public on the high quality of the care provided by the NHS.

- Stay ahead – by introducing new treatments that permit the care provided to be labelled as high-quality care. Supporting innovation was also a cornerstone of the review.

ACTIVITY 9.2

Reflection: Why do you think that 'quality in health care' is now a paramount priority of health care professionals? How would you 'translate' the previous steps to public health interventions beyond health care contexts?

Measuring quality

Measuring quality in health care and public health interventions can be challenging as the very definition of what is quality varies among different stakeholders. For example, service users or customers review quality as service responsiveness to cater to their interests and needs; practitioners often link quality with available health services as well as adequate human capacities to manage public needs and interests at an appropriate level; whereas donors or commissioners conceptualise quality as the extent to which there is rational utilisation of funds or resources (Clarke and Rao, 2004).

It can be claimed, however, that in general there are ways of measuring quality health care using the structure within which the care is provided, the process of delivering the service care and the outcomes of the services (Rillon, 2000, page 291). This approach is also called Donabedian's (1980) 'structure and process approach' which has been viewed as a holistic approach in measuring quality of health care.

Structure

Structure refers to the degree to which the care system will be planned and delivered, and the resources that are available. Rillon (2000, page 291) claims that this is the easiest aspect compared with those two, but still this aspect has not been dealt with properly. Some aspects of structure are:

- facilities – comforts, convenience of layout, accessibility of support services and safety;
- equipment – adequate supplies, state of the art equipment and staff capacity to use them;
- staff – credentials, experience, absenteeism, turnover rate, service provider–user ratios; and
- finance – salaries, adequacy and resources.

Process

This is concerned with the actual public health activities or interventions carried out by the health service practitioners; for example, this could be identification and recognition of problems, diagnostic procedures (health needs assessment); access to, and utilisation and management of, health services. This also includes psychological interventions, for example, teaching and counselling, as well as physical care measures.

Outcome

This refers to the results of the health activities or interventions in which the health service providers have been primarily involved and engaged. It can also be defined as changes in users' health status, including their expectations and satisfaction with the care provided.

Standards in these aspects are formulated as a basis of comparison in the assessment of quality, such as in the structure and process as well as outcomes of care which exist. Standards vary depending upon the level of implementation and the procedures used in collecting data/information, and depending on the aim of the programme and the intended outcome.

The NHS approach

In the UK, the 'High Quality Care for All' review situated the task of measuring quality as one of the main steps in quality improvement (Department of Health–NHS, 2008, page 48) because, as Lord Darzi stated, 'We can only be sure to improve what we can actually measure' (Department of Health–NHS, 2008, page 49). The theoretical framework used by NHS for quality improvement (Figure 9.1) describes how the process of quality improvement should operate.

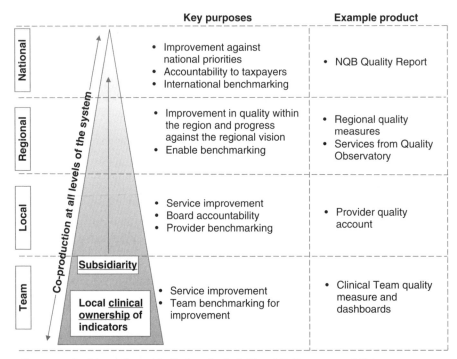

Figure 9.1 Quality pyramid overview of the quality indicators framework.

The framework for measuring quality in the NHS starts from the bottom of the pyramid or the forefront of the service delivery – the teams of both health professionals and all those who support them – as those responsible for the lead and delivery of high-quality services. At this level the strategy focuses on supporting teams for data collection and analysis and for their own development of improvement skills.

In the same line, local teams and organisations are free to choose the metrics they need to measure quality of services internally but demands that they are supported by the relevant measures for benchmarking regionally and nationally.

The NHS strategy gives the teams the freedom to choose indicators and to decide priorities for quality improvement but demands the continuous and systematic collection of data to ensure informed practice and innovation. From them, it works upwards.

At regional level, the strategy sees the Strategic Health Authorities' (SHAs) role as those able to measure overall improvement on some key measures and account for the quality of care delivered while providing support and coordination so the measurement and improvement is coherent across systems.

Finally, at national level, a small core set of metrics covering the three dimensions of quality – patient safety, patient experience and effectiveness of treatment – should be used to measure progress against national priorities and to allow international comparisons (NHS, 2009b, page 2).

The framework also articulates the principles for change as (NHS, 2009b, page 2).

- Co-production – implementation should be discussed and decided in partnership with the NHS, local authorities and key stakeholders.

- Subsidiarity: where necessary, the centre will play an enabling role, but the priority is that the implementation details are decided at local level.

- Clinical ownership and leadership: NHS staff will be active participants and leaders of the process of quality improvement.

- System alignment: the whole system must be aligned to the same aim (the improvement of quality) while allowing the use of the combined leverage at every level.

Indicators for quality improvement (IQI)

Following the declaration of the three dimensions of quality – patient safety, patient experience and effectiveness of treatment – a set of indicators to measure quality improvement has been developed. The indicators for quality improvement (IQI) are meant to be a resource for local clinical teams in their selection of indicators for quality improvement, a source for benchmarking, a set of indicators granted with the credibility of been assured by clinicians – and therefore suited for the purpose of being used by clinicians – and a transparent source of information since they are published with full metada. (In the current IQI (version 21) metadata items are provided for each indicator. Metadata explain the methodology and data sources used and link to the original indicator source of the calculated indicators.)

The current version is a list of 200 IQIs with an extra 50 having been developed and therefore the full display of the list exceeds the limits of this chapter. An example of indicators in each of the quality dimensions is presented in Table 9.1 (NHS, 2010).

Table 9.1 Examples of indicators for quality improvement (IQIs)

Ref. no.	Title	Quality dimension	NSR pathway
CV35	Percentage of ST-elevation myocardial infarction (STEMI) patients who received primary angioplasty within 120 minutes of call (call to balloon time)	Effectiveness	Acute Care
WCC 2.09	Proportion of children who complete MMR immunisation by 2nd birthday	Effectiveness	Children's health
CA45	Proportion of incident cases reviewed by multidisciplinary team (MDT) for all cancers	Effectiveness	Planned care
PE49	Score for patients who reported that the hospital room or ward was very or fairly clean	Patient experience	Other
PE41	Score for patients who reported that they always or sometimes had confidence and trust in the doctors treating them	Patient experience	Other
PE16	Score for patients who reported that they were involved as much as they wanted to be in decisions about their care and treatment	Patient experience	Other
PS39	Incidence of MRSA bacteraemia	Safety	Planned care
NRSL3	Rate of patient safety events occurring in trusts that were submitted to the Reporting and Learning System (RLS)	Safety	Planned care
PS15	Medicines – acute trusts compliant with safety standards – Care Quality Commission's Annual Health Check data	Safety	Planned care

Source: Adapted from NHS. The Information Centre for Health and Social Care (2009a).

Effectiveness

The concept of effectiveness in health care has evolved dramatically from its first conceptions – used to refer to the extent a treatment or drug produces the expected effects – to the more modern one that includes the assessment of a wide range of parameters to measure the quality of health care. For instance, NHS Scotland defines clinical effectiveness as a group of quality improvement activities and initiatives including (NHS Scotland, 2007):

- Evidence, guidelines and standards to identify and implement best practice

- Quality improvement tools (clinical audit, evaluation, rapid cycle improvement) used for the review and improvement of treatments and services.

Such tools take into consideration the views of patients, service users and staff, evidence from incidents, near-misses, clinical risks and risk analysis, outcomes from treatments or services, and measurement service/department's performance against set-up goals:

- identifying areas for further research;

- as information systems aiming to assess current practice and including the search for evidence of improvement;

- assessing of the cost-effectiveness of services/treatments;

- developing and using of organisational learning systems.

As we discussed early in this chapter the importance and intimate relationship between quality and effectiveness is made clear by the 'High Quality Care for All' framework NHS document (Department of Health–NHS, 2008, page 33) that places effectiveness as one of the three dimensions of quality.

There are many indexes of clinical effectiveness. Some, such as the Cochrane Library, have been covered in earlier chapters; but other search engines and databases include the Turning Research into Practice (TRIP) database (a free access search database that covers a wide range of UK and US clinical effectiveness resources) and the Database of Abstracts of Reviews of Effects (DARE), part of the Centre for Reviews and Dissemination-National Institute for Health Research (NIHR), University of York that focuses on the effects of interventions used in health and social care.

The differences between clinical effectiveness and public health effectiveness are not clear, with the main areas of difference found in the scope of the analysis performed. Thus, in assessing effectiveness in public health, efforts are directed to the analysis of interventions and campaigns aimed at improving the health of the population as a whole. To illustrate the case and to conclude this section we offer a case study.

Case study 9.1: Effectiveness of nurse home visits to primarious mothers and infants

Nurse home visits are believed to be an important tool for the delivery of public health nursing services. They have many advantages (e.g. convenient for family, client-controlled setting, facilitates access to care when there are transport problems, for example, and so on). However it is a very expensive service and its effectiveness on the promotion of health during the childbearing and early postpartum periods was in doubt. In 1983, Violet H Barkauskas published the findings from a study aimed at determining the effects of public health nurse postpartum home visits in a county in a Midwestern State in the USA. She interviewed two groups of randomly selected mothers–children (67 had received nurse home visits and 43 had not received them) using a postpartum interview questionnaire (PIQ) and Home Observation for Measurement of the Environment (HOME) tool. Her effectiveness measures were 18 variables surveying mother's health and health services utilisation, infant's health and health services utilisation, and mother's parenting practices. Her statistical analysis (mainly multivariate contingency table and two-way analysis of variance techniques) revolved around whether there were differences in the scores obtained in those questionnaires among women who had received home nurse visits and women who had not. She found that only one variable demonstrated significant public health home visit nursing effect: home-visited mothers were more apt to express concerns about health matters than not-home-visited mothers.

Barkauskas' study provided evidence that home visits were not more effective in achieving general health promotion goals among primarious mothers compared to services provided for the same goal in health centres. Taking into account the costs there was little argument supporting continuation and funding of such services. Her study, however, also included the perception of mothers on the usefulness of such visits and the findings were clear: women believed such visits had been useful.

(Based on Barkauskas, 1983)

ACTIVITY 9.3

More than 20 years after the study described in Case study 9.1, nurse home visits continue to be standard practice for mothers in most western countries. The case study invites reflections on why evidence of effectiveness has been disregarded. Discuss in small groups:

- Have other (newer, stronger) studies contradicted these findings? How would you answer this question?
- If postpartum nurse home visits have been sustained in consideration of clients' perceptions, what are the implications regarding the value and suitability of effectiveness analysis?

Clinical audit: a tool for quality improvement

Another of the concepts close to quality is audit. In this chapter we provide a summary overview of the concept and its main mechanism. Defining 'audit' is not a simple task as the term is applied widely to different areas of health care and it has many other related concepts. Thus while management audit and clinical audit seem to be the main two types of audits, terms such as 'care pathways', 'performance evaluation', 'programme evaluation' and 'quality assurance' are closely related to audit activities. It is important to remember, however, that both audit and quality assurance aim to provide evidence, and it is important to include such concepts in a book such as this one concerned with public health evidence.

The most common type of audit in health care is the clinical audit because clinical audits are necessary for the assessment of the quality of care provided. Other tools under this remit include patient experience surveys, critical incident enquiries and research with qualitative methods.

The widely accepted definition of clinical audit was produced by the National Institute for Health and Clinical Excellence (NICE), the Commission for Health Improvement (CHI) and the Royal College of Nursing (RCN) and it defines the concept as: 'Clinical audit is a quality improvement process that seeks to improve patient care and outcomes through systematic review of care against explicit criteria and the implementation of change' (2009, page 2).

But a recent initiative of the National Clinical Audit Advisory Group (NCAAG) has been to produce a definition of the concept in accordance to its modern understanding:

> *Clinical audit is the assessment of the process (using evidence-based criteria) and/or the outcome of care (by comparison with others). Its aim is to stimulate and support national and local quality improvement interventions and, through re-auditing, to assess the impact of such interventions.*
>
> (Black, 2009, page 2)

Audits are strategic tools for governance and their importance was fully acknowledged when the 2000 NHS Plan (Department of Health, 2009) made it mandatory for all doctors to participate in clinical audits.

From what we have written so far it is clear that clinical audit implies the use of a set of broad methods drawn from different disciplines (e.g. organisational development, statistics and information management) aiming to assess a clinical scenario and detect potential sources of improvement.

Although the complete dissection of audit types and methodologies goes beyond the scope of this chapter (see Going further section for suggestions on further reading) the general model has been described as a five-step process – preparing for the audit, selecting criteria, measuring performance, making improvements and sustaining improvement. This can be applied to the clinical situation to be audited. The general cycle of an audit is presented in Figure 9.2.

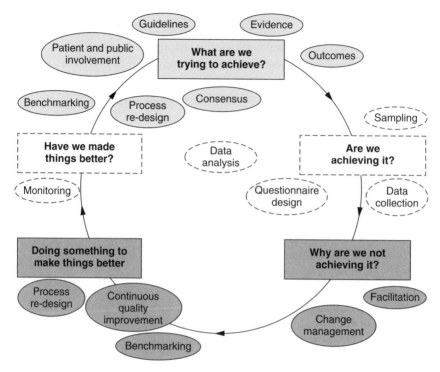

Figure 9.2 The clinical audit cycle.

Source: National Institute for Clinical Excellence (2002, page 3).

Chapter summary

In this chapter we started with the concept of quality and quality in health care and we introduced you to the dimensions of quality care and their roles in making public health services more effective. We also discussed some key features of quality and ways of assessing them in health care:

- Use of different types/areas of quality and evidence and translation of quality evidence into public health practices – what it is used for?
- Quality improvement strategies (using an example of NHS)
- Measuring quality improvements – tools, indicators, clinical auditing, including structure and outcomes framework
- Evaluating quality and its effectiveness in public health programmes.

- The Quality Care Commission www.cqc.org.uk
  This is an independent regulator of health and social care quality in England. It regulates care provided by the NHS, local authorities, private companies and voluntary organisations.

- The European Society of Quality in Health Care
  www.esqh.net/newsfolder_view?portal_status_title=ESQH+NEWS
  This website is the virtual tool of the European Society of Quality in Health Care (ESQH) dedicated to the improvement of quality in European health care among 20 EU member states, including the UK.

- Archive of 'Quality in Health Care' www.ncbi.nlm.nih.gov/pmc/journals/175
  This is an essential website (archive) for those who are interested in learning quality and quality in health care.

Conclusion
Carmen Aceijas

At the beginning of this book we quoted Jenicek's definition of evidence-based public health:

> *the conscientious explicit and judicious use of current best evidence in making decisions about the care of communities and populations in the domain of health protection, disease prevention, health maintenance and improvement.*
>
> (Jenicek, 1997, pages 187–197)

Throughout the nine chapters the different contributing authors have offered concepts, descriptions, explanations, case studies and activities to help the reader in the quest of evidence in a variety of public health contexts.

Chapter 1 covers a generic introduction to the subject, enabling readers to identify the nature and main features of evidence-based public health, to be aware of the origins of the concept, to understand the different key aspects of evidence-based public health, and to become familiar with the basic process of gathering information and assessing evidence.

Thus, the key features and aims of evidence-based public health – conceptual plausibility, use of different types of evidence and translation of evidence into practical guidance for policy and practice – and the contexts where evidence-based public health is especially needed – when scientific evidence must support decision making, to evaluate the effectiveness and cost benefits of public health programmes, to implement new public health programmes or interventions, when new policies must be established, to conduct literature reviews for grant projects – are discussed.

The chapter also allows the identification of the benefits that the evidence-based public health approach has brought to public health. Some of the most important ones are that it enables the decision-making processes to be based on scientific evidence and effective practices, it facilitates the retrieval of up-to-date and reliable information about what works and does not work for a given public health issue and it provides reassurance on the efficiency of public health measures.

Finally, we present a practical introduction to the process of gathering information via a seven-step module and critical appraisal, allowing students to start to see how the conceptual contents translate in practice.

Chapter 2 is an excellent tool to learn how to search for information applicable to public health. It includes an introduction to the Cochrane Collaboration – an invaluable source of evidence in public health – and provides comprehensive guidance on database searching techniques using search engines and databases such MEDLINE,

Embase, CINAHL, PsycINFO, DARE and Trip Database. It also introduces information services relevant to our discipline, such as the CenterWatch clinical trials listing services and the British Library EThOS (Electronic Theses Online Service).

One of the features of this chapter is its step-by-step approach to demonstrate how to search for information. The student is presented with different tools such as keywords and Boolean searching, combining words, phrase searching, truncation/wildcard searching that will help to systematise and improve the efficiency of his or her search.

The chapter includes not only 'mechanical guidelines' on how to search for information but also a dissection of the designs and aspects of studies, such as reliability and validity, which must to be taken into account when assessing the strength of evidence generated. This added value enables the reader to go much further than the plain retrieval of information.

Chapter 3 presents the well-known model of hierarchy of evidence, a tool for decision making that uses the design of studies with classificatory aims. There, the relationship between a study's research design and the level or strength of research evidence emerging from the research studies was explored. In this model, five levels of evidence are considered: Level I-1: a systematic review and/or meta-analyses, Level I-2: an RCT, Level II-1: a cohort design, Level II-2: a case–control design, Level II-3: a cross-sectional design, Level II-4: a case series design, Level III: well-designed non-experimental studies and Levels IV and V professional or expert opinion and 'someone told me . . .'. Rather than focusing on a full description of every design (which would be more appropriate for a different kind of volume), the chapter presents their main characteristics and the arguments for their location in the hierarchy of evidence. The chapter also includes descriptions of how to use the model and reflections on the limits of such hierarchy.

Chapter 4 offers an in-depth examination of the process of critical appraisal as a careful and systematic process, and is focused on judging the 'trustworthiness' and relevance of research evidence to practice (Burls, 2009, page 1). The chapter gives a comprehensive description of the steps and tools available to conduct critical appraisal of public health literature. The author reminds us of the importance of the basics a good reviewer must have (e.g. able to read scientific literature, able to search for scientific literature) before embarking on a appraisal task. The chapter includes insightful suggestions for the selection of the appraisal tool and extensive information on how to present the findings from an appraisal by building robust and credible arguments. Finally it offers reflective arguments on the most common errors found in appraisal exercises.

Chapter 5 deals with issues surrounding the assessment of evidence from primary and secondary sources. The preoccupation with the quality expected from the two main types of research (and the specific designs that are grouped under the two remits) is important and remains controversial. The authors of this chapter provide an insightful overview of the concept of quality in research and how the debate is presented when analysing information found in secondary and primary sources. The presentation of GRADE (Grading of Recommendation Assessment, Development and Evaluation) as a system to judge evidence from different research designs is a well-thought out option for those aiming to learn the use of systematic tools officially endorsed and adopted by numerous organisations for this purpose. The chapter also includes a number of activities and exercises that help the readers to learn and practise skills to assess quality of evidence.

Chapter 6 introduces the reader to a different kind of use of evidence-based public health, which focuses on assessing programmes and the effectiveness of public health interventions rather than on pure research. In this line the chapter acknowledges that evaluation or assessment is a basic function of management but the document goes much further than that and examines the concept of evidence from the viewpoint of the patients/service users, or policy makers, and ways of assessing evidence in health care interventions. With a very clear practical aim in mind, the author provides an eclectic array of ideas and concepts and introduces us to some models and tools for the assessment of programmes that facilitate a first approach to programme assessments by the reader. Chapter 6 is clearly linked to Chapter 8 as they share the same main focus: how to ascertain the evidence regarding the impact of programmes and interventions in public health.

Chapter 7 addresses the important issue of including economic factors when assessing evidence. In these times of financial hardship and as awareness of the importance of assessment on how economically sound findings of public health programmes and interventions are, the contents of this chapter become especially relevant. In this chapter the author's commitment was to help students to learn how to set priorities on the basis of evidence-based public health. The chapter opens the subject with an introduction to cost-effectiveness analysis but it is especially focused on the gold standard: cost–utility ratio calculation of public health interventions. For that purpose the chapter uses a scaffolding model to guide the reader through the learning processes of estimating savings in averted treatment costs as a result of morbidity decreases caused by the intervention, estimating increased quality-adjusted life years (QALYs) due to morbidity reductions caused by the intervention and estimating increased QALYs due to mortality reductions caused by the intervention. The chapter aims to introduce some main concepts and tools in economic assessment of public health interventions, allowing the reader to approach more specialised health economics literature.

Chapter 8 focuses exclusively on the evaluation of programmes and in this sense should be read in connection with Chapter 6. It thoroughly explores and dissects the framework for evaluation of public health programmes endorsed by the Centers for Disease Control (CDC) step by step: Step 1: engage stakeholders, Step 2: describe the programme, Step 3: focus the evaluation design, Step 4: gather credible evidence, Step 5: justify conclusions and Step 6: ensure use and share lessons learned. The chapter is especially careful to make students aware of the activities and points for consideration at every step, from the definition of stakeholders to the outline of the evaluation design and the main available data collection methods and including the development of the logic model and set of indicators to be used without leaving out the latest steps of the framework, which include communication of the findings and follow-up activities.

Finally, Chapter 9 introduces the reader to several concepts related to quality in public health. The aims of this chapter are to critically understand the concept of quality and its role in public health and health care, discuss some tools and measures of quality and effectiveness, reflect on the relationships between quality and effectiveness and understand the role of audit as a quality improvement tool. These are all fulfilled by descriptive descriptions of concepts and tools used in this area and activities to illustrate practical applications. The NHS approach to quality is described in this chapter and an acknowledgement made of the leadership role that the 'High Quality Care for All' review has provided (Department of Health–NHS, 2008), including the expertise created and sustained by this organisation in the area of quality assurance and improvement in health services in general and in public health in particular.

All nine chapters aim to build the expertise needed among current and future public health advanced practitioners and specialists as defined by the Department of Health in the PHSCF (Department of Health–NHS, 2008). Hence, a capacity-building approach directed the objectives in deciding the contents of this volume and aims to guarantee that our discipline remains as:

> the science and art of preventing disease, prolonging life and promoting mental and physical health through organised efforts of society.
>
> (Acheson, 1988)

References

Abrams, P (1985) The uses of British sociology, in Mulner, M (ed.) *Essay on the History of British Sociological Research*. Cambridge: Cambridge University Press.

Acheson, D (1988) *Public Health in England*. London: Department of Health.

Alkin, M (1997) Stakeholder concepts in programme evaluation, in Reynolds, A and Wallberg, H (eds) *Evaluation for Educational Productivity*. Greenwich, CT: JAI.

Atkins, D, Eccles, M, Flottorp, S, Guyatt, G, Henry, D, Hill, S and the GRADE Working Group (2004) Systems for grading the quality of evidence and the strength of recommendations I: Critical appraisal of existing approaches. *BMC Health Services Research*, 4: 38.

Barbour, R (2001) Checklists for improving rigour in qualitative research: a case of the tail wagging dog? *British Medical Journal*, 322: 115–117.

Barkauskas, VH (1983) Effectiveness of public health nurse home visits to primarous mothers and their infants. *American Journal of Public Health*, 73: 573–580.

Batty, G, Shipley, M, Gunnell, D, Smith, G, Ferrie, J, Clarke, R *et al.* (2010) Height loss and future coronary heart disease in London: the Whitehall II study. *Journal of Epidemiology and Community Health*, 30 [E-pub ahead of print].

Baum, F (2010) *The New Public Health*, 3rd edition. Oxford: Oxford University Press.

Bestall, JC, Paul, EA, Garrod, RA, Garnham, R, Jones, PW and Wedzicha, JA (1999) Usefulness of the Medical Council (MRC) dyspnoea scale as a measure of disability in patients with chronic obstructive pulmonary disease. *Thorax* 54: 581–586.

Black, N (2009) Publications, policy and guidance. 'What is clinical audit?' NCAAG, Department of Health, 8 October 2009. www.dh.gov.uk/en/Publicationsandstatistics/Publications/PublicationsPolicyAndGuidance/DH_103396?ssSourceSiteId=ab (accessed 22 October 2010).

Borgerson, K (2009) Valuing evidence: bias and the evidence hierarchy of evidence-based medicine. *Perspectives in Biological Medicine*, 52: 218–233.

Boyle, AH and Locke, DL (2004) Update on chronic obstructive pulmonary disease. *Medsurg Nursing*, 13: 42–48.

Brown, P, Brunnhuber, K, Chalkidou, K, Chalmers, I, Clarke, M, Fenton, M *et al.* (2006) Health research. How to formulate research recommendations. *British Medical Journal*, 333: 804–806.

Brownson, RC, Gurney, JG and Land, GH (1999) Evidence-based decision making in public health. *Journal of Public Health Management Practice*, 5: 86–97.

Brownson, RC, Baker, EA, Leet, TL and Gillespie, KN (eds) (2003) *Evidence-Based Public Health*. New York: Oxford University Press.

Burls, A (2009) *What is Critical Appraisal?* London: Hayward Medical Communications.

Campbell, D and Stanley, J (1963) *Experimental and Quasi-experimental Designs for Research*. Chicago: Rand McNally College Publishing.

Canadian Taskforce on the Periodic Health Examination (1979) The periodic health examination. *Canadian Medical Association Journal*, 121: 1193–1254.

Carr, A, Unwin, N and Pless-Mulloli, T (2007) *An Introduction to Public Health and Epidemiology*. Maidenhead: Open University Press.

Centre for Reviews and Dissemination (CRD) (2009) *Systematic Reviews: CDR's guidance for undertaking reviews in health care*. York: CRD.

Centers for Disease Control and Prevention (CDC) (1999) Framework for program evaluation in public health. *Morbidity and Mortality Weekly Report*, 48(RR11): 1–40.

Centers for Disease Control and Prevention (CDC) (2010) Use of a self-assessment questionnaire for food safety education in the home kitchen. Los Angeles County, California, 2006–2008. *Morbidity and Mortality Weekly Report*, 59(34): 1098–1101.

Chelimsky, E (1995) Where we stand today in the practice of evaluation. *Knowledge and Policy*, 8: 8–19.

Ciliska, D, Thomas, H and Buffett, C (2008) *A Compendium of Critical Appraisal Tools for Public Health Practice*. Hamilton, ON: National Collaborating Centre for Methods and Tools (NCCMT).

Clarke, A and Rao, M (2004) Developing quality indicators to assess quality of care. *Quality and Safety in Health Care*, 13: 248–249.

Cochrane, AL (1972) *Effectiveness and Efficiency: Random Reflections on Health Services*. London: British Medical Journal/Nuffield Provincial Hospital Trust.

Cochrane, AL (1979) 1931–1971: a critical review, with particular reference to the medical profession, in Feeling-Smith, G and Wells, N (eds) *Medicines for the Year 2000*. London: Office of Health Economics.

Crombie, I (1996) *The Pocket Guide To Critical Appraisal*. London: BMJ Publishing.

Crombie, I (2007) *The Pocket Guide to Critical Appraisal*, 2nd revised edition. London: Wiley-Blackwell.

Crouch, R, Buckley, R and Fenton, K (2003) Consultant nurses: the next generation. *Emergency Nurse*, 11(7): 15–17.

Dahlberg, L and McCaig, C (2010) *Practical Research and Evaluation: A start-to-finish guide for practitioners*. London: Sage.

Daly, J, Willis, K, Small, R, Green, J, Welch, N, Kealy, M and Hughes, E (2007) A hierarchy of evidence for assessing qualitative health research. *Journal of Clinical Epidemiology*, 60: 43–49.

Das, K, Malick, S, and Khan, KS (2008) Tips for teaching evidence-based medicine in a clinical setting: lessons from adult learning theory. Part one. *Journal of the Royal Society of Medicine*, 101: 493–500.

Del Mar, C, Glasziou, P and Mayer, D (2004) Teaching evidence-based medicine. *British Medical Journal*, 329: 989–990.

Department of Health (2008) *UK Public Health Skills and Career Framework: Multidisciplinary/multi-agency/multi-professional*. London: Department of Health, Public Health Resource Unit, Skills for Health. www.sph.nhs.uk/sph-files/PHSkills-CareerFramework_Launchdoc_April08.pdf (accessed April 2011).

Department of Health (2009) *Publications, Policy and Guidance*. 'What is Clinical Audit?' Nick Black Chair, NCAAG. 8 October 2009. www.dh.gov.uk/en/Publicationsandstatistics/Publications/PublicationsPolicyAndGuidance/DH_103396?ssSourceSiteId=ab (accessed 22 October 2010).

Department of Health (2010) *Healthy Life, Healthy People: Our Strategy for Public Health in England*. London: Department of Health.

Department of Health–NHS (2008) *High Quality Care for All: NHS Next Stage Review Final Report*. London: Department of Health.

Department of Health–NHS (2010) *Equity and Excellence: Liberating the NHS*. London: Department of Health.

Donabedian, A (1980) The definition of quality: a conceptual exploration, in: *Exploration in Quality Assessment and Monitoring*. Vol. I: *The definition of quality and approaches to its assessment*. Ann Arbor, MI: Health Administration Press.

Dyal, WW (1995) Ten organizational practices of public health: a historical perspective. *American Journal of Preventive Medicine*, 11(Suppl 2): 6–8.

Ewles, L and Simnett, I (2010) *Promoting Health: A Practical Guide*. London: Baillière Tindall.

Fajo-Pascual, M, Godoy, P, Ferro-cancer, M and Wymore, K (2010) Case-control study of risk factors for sporadic Campylobacter infection in northeastern Spain. *European Journal of Public Health*, 20: 443–448.

Fritsche, L, Greenhalgh, T, Falck-Ytter, Y, Neumayer, K and Kunz, R (2002) Do short courses in evidence-based medicine improve knowledge and skills? Validation of Berlin questionnaire and before and after study of courses in evidence-based medicine. *British Medical Journal*, 325: 1338–1341.

Gagne, RM, Bridges, LJ and Wagne, WW (1998) *Principles of Instructional Design*. Orlando, FL: Holt, Rinehart and Winston, Inc.

Gersten, R, Baker, S, and Lloyd, JW (2000) Designing high-quality research in special education: group experimental design. *Journal of Special Education*, 34(1): 2–18.

Gillam, S, Yates, J and Badrinath, P (2007) *Essential Public Health: Theory and Practice*. Cambridge: Cambridge University Press.

Ginsberg, GM (2003) Internal working paper, WHO, VAM.

Ginsberg, G, Fisher, M, Ben-Shahar, I and Bornstein, J (2007) Cost utility analysis of vaccination against HPV in Israel. *Vaccine*, 25: 6677–6691.

Ginsberg, GM, Lim, S, Lauer, JA, Johns, BP and Sepulveda, CR (2010a) Prevention, screening and treatment of colorectal cancer: a global and regional generalized cost effectiveness analysis. *Cost Effectiveness and Resource Allocation*, 8: 2. www.resource-allocation.com/content/8/1/2 (accessed 3 January 2011).

Ginsberg, G, Rosen, B and Rosenberg, E (2010b) Cost-utility analyses of interventions to reduce the smoking-related burden of disease in Israel. RR-540-10. Brookdale-Smokler Centre for health policy research. http://brookdale.jdc. org.il/?CategoryID=192&ArticleID=115 (accessed 10 October 2010).

Girden, E (1996) *Evaluating Research Articles: From Start to Finish*. Thousand Oaks, CA: Sage.

Goldie, SJ, O'Shea, M, Campos, NG, Dias, M, Sweet, S and Kim, SY (2008) Health and economic outcomes of HPV 16,18 vaccination in 72 GAVI-eligible countries. *Vaccine*, 26: 4080–4093.

Green, ML (1999) Graduate medical education training in clinical epidemiology, critical appraisal and evidence-based medicine: a critical review of curricula. *Academic Medicine*, 74: 686–694.

Greenhalgh, T (2004) *How to Read a Paper*, 2nd edition. London: BMJ Publishing.

Greenhalgh, T (2006) *How to Read a Paper: The Basics of Evidence-based Medicine*, 3rd edn. Oxford: Blackwell Publishing.

Guyatt, G and Drummond, R (2002) *User's Guides to the Medical Literature: A Manual for Evidence-Based Practice*. Chicago: American Medical Association.

Guyton, AC and Hall, JE (2000) *Textbook of Medical Physiology*. Philadelphia: WB Saunders Elsevier: 9–12.

Handler, AS, Turnock, BJ and Hall, W (1995) A strategy for measuring local public health practice. *American Journal of Preventive Medicine*, 11(6): 29–35.

Handler, A, Issel, M and Turnock, B (2001) A conceptual framework to measure performance of the public health system. *American Journal of Public Health*, 91(8): 1235–1239.

Hatala, R and Guyatt, G (2002) Evaluating the teaching of evidence-based medicine. *Journal of the American Medical Association*, 288: 1110–1112.

Heller, R, Verma, A, Gemmell, I, Harrison, R, Hart, J and Edwards, R (2008) Critical appraisal for public health: a new checklist. *Public Health*, 122(1): 92–98.

Hennink, MM (2007) *International Focus Group Research*. Cambridge: Cambridge University Press.

Higgins, JPT and Deeks, JJ (2008) Chapter 7: Selecting studies and collecting data, in Higgins, JPT and Green, S (eds) *Cochrane Handbook for Systematic Reviews of Interventions*. Version 5.0.0. The Cochrane Collaboration. Available from: www.cochrane-handbook.org.

Holland, W (1983) *Evaluation of Health Care*. Oxford: Oxford University Press.

House, ER (1978, 1986) *New Directions in Educational Evaluation*. London: Falmer Press.

Ilic, D (2009) Assessing competency in evidence-based practice: strengths and limitations of current tools in practice. *BMC Medical Education*, 9: 53.

Jenicek, M (1997) Epidemiology, evidence-based medicine, and evidence-based public health. *Journal of Epidemiology*, 7: 187–197.

Jenkinson, C (1997) *Assessment and Evaluation of Health and Medical Care: A Methods Text*. Maidenhead: Open University Press.

Jewell, EJ and Abate, F (eds) (2001) *The New Oxford American Dictionary*. New York: Oxford University Press.

Joint Committee on Standards for Educational Evaluation (1994) *Program Evaluation Standards: How to Assess Evaluations of Educational Programs*, 2nd edition. Thousand Oaks, CA: Sage Publications.

Killoran, A and Kelly, MP (2010) Introduction: effectiveness and efficiency in public health, in *Evidence Based Public Health. Effectiveness and Efficiency*. Oxford: Oxford University Press.

Knapp, MS (1996) Methodological issues in evaluating integrated services initiatives, in Marquart, JM and Konrad, EL (eds) *Evaluating Initiatives to Integrate Human Services*. San Francisco: Jossey-Bass Publishers, pp.21–34

Koplan, JP (1999) CDC sets millennium priorities. *US Medicine*, 4–7.

Lincoln, Y and Guba, E (1985) *Naturalistic Inquiry*. Beverly Hills, CA: Sage.

Locke, DL and Boyle, AH (2002) Patient advocacy: a multi-disciplinary mandate, in Hedrick, HL and Kutscher, AH (eds) *The Quiet Killer: Emphysema/chronic Obstructive Pulmonary Disease*. Lanham, MD: Scarecrow Press, pp.199–204.

Lockett, T (1997) *Evidence-Based and Cost-Effective Medicine for the Unintended*. Oxford and New York: Radcliff Medical Press.

Makela, M and Witt, K (2005) How to read a paper: critical appraisal of studies for application in health care. *Singapore Medical Journal*, 46(3): 108–114.

Maxwell, RJ (1992) Quality assessment in health. *British Medical Journal*, 288: 1470–1472.

Mays, GP, Halverson, PK and Miller, CA (1998) Assessing the performance of local public health systems: a survey of state health agency efforts. *Journal of Public Health Manage Practice*, 4(4): 63–78.

McNamara, C (2000) Basic guide to program evaluation. www.managementhelp.org/evaluatn/fnl_eval.htm#anchor1585345 (accessed 25 October 2010).

McQueen, DV and Anderson, LM (2001) What counts as evidence? Issues and debates, in Rootman, I (ed.) *Evaluation in Health Promotion: Principles and Perspectives*. Copenhagen, Denmark: World Health Organization, pp.63–81.

Mella, MP, Maligat, RA and Yanga-Mabunga, ST (2000) *Programme or Project Evaluation*. Manila: UPM.

Miller, CA, Moore, KS, Richards, TB and McKaig, C (1994b) A screening survey to assess local public health performance. *Public Health Repository*, 109: 659–664.

Miller, CA, Moore, KS, Richards, TB and Monk, JD (1994a) A proposed method for assessing the performance of local public health functions and practices. *American Journal of Public Health*, 84: 1743–1749.

Miller, G (1990) The assessment of clinical skills/competence/performance. *Academic Medicine*, 129: 42–48.

Mosteller, F and Boruch, R (eds) (2002) *Evidence Matters: Randomized Trials in Education Research*. Washington, DC: The Brookings Institute.

Naidoo, J and Wills, J (forthcoming) *Health Promotion and Practice: Developing an Evidence Base*. London: Elsevier.

NICE (National Institute for Health and Clinical Excellence) (2002) *Principles for Best Practice in Clinical Audit*. Abingdon: Radcliffe Medical Press.

NICE (2004) National clinical guideline management of chronic obstructive pulmonary disease in adults primary and secondary care. *Thorax*, 59(Suppl 1): S1–232.

NCDDR (National Center for the Dissemination of Disability Research) (2003) Evidence-based research in education. *The Research Exchange*, 8(2): 16.

Neuman, WL (2006) *Social Research Methods: Quantitative and Qualitative Approaches*. Boston: Pearson Education.

NHS (1996) *Promoting Clinical Effectiveness: A Framework for Action in and Through the NHS*. Leeds: Department of Health.

NHS (2000a) The Information Centre for Health and Social Care. Quality pyramid. www.ic.nhs.uk/webfiles/Work%20with%20us/consultations/CQI/QualityPyramid.pdf (accessed 21 October 2010).

NHS (2009b) The Information Centre for Health and Social Care. High quality care for all – measuring for quality improvement: the approach. www.ic.nhs.uk/webfiles/Work%20with%20us/consultations/CQI/MeasuringforQualityImprovement%20_2_.pdf (accessed 21 October 2010).

NHS (2010) The Information Centre for Health and Social Care. Indicators for quality improvement. Full indicators list. https://mqi.ic.nhs.uk/ (accessed 21 October 2010).

NHS Scotland (2007) What is clinical effectiveness? NHS Scotland. Education Sources. Clinical Governance. www.clinicalgovernance.scot.nhs.uk/section2/clinicaleffectiveness.asp (accessed April 2011).

Norman, G and Shannon, S (1998) Effectiveness of instruction in critical appraisal skills: a critical appraisal. *Canadian Medical Association Journal*, 158: 177–181.

Oliver, S and Peersman, G (2001) Critical appraisal of research evidence: finding useful and reliable answers, in Oliver, S and Peersman, G (eds) *Using Research for Effective Health Promotion*. Buckingham: Open University Press, pp.82–95.

Patton, MQ (1982) *Practical Evaluation*. Beverley Hills, CA: Sage.

Patton, MQ (2002) *Qualitative Research and Evaluation Methods*. London: Sage.

Pawson, R and Sridharan, S (2010) Theory-driven evaluation of public health programmes, in Killoran, A and Kelly, MP (eds) *Evidence-Based Public Health: Effectiveness and Efficiency*. Oxford: Oxford University Press, p.49.

Pawson, R and Tilley, N (1997) *Realistic Evaluation*. London: Sage Publications.

Petticrew, M and Roberts, H (2003) Evidence, hierarchies and typologies: horses for courses. *Journal of Epidemiology and Community Health*, 57: 527–529.

Pisani, E (2008) *The Wisdom of Whores: Bureaucrats, Brothels and the Business of AIDS*. London: Granta.

Public Health Resource Unit (2010) www.phru.nhs.uk (accessed 22 November 2010).

Ramos, K, Schafer, S and Tracz, V (2003) Validation of the Fresno test of competence in evidence based medicine. *British Medical Journal*, 326: 319–321.

Regmi, K, Naidoo, J, Pilkington, P and Greer, A (2010) Decentralization and district health services in Nepal: understanding the views of service users and service providers. *Journal of Public Health*, 32(3): 406–417.

Richards, TB, Rogers, JJ, Christenson, GM, Miller, CA and Gatewood, DD (1995a) Assessing public health practice: application of ten core function measures of community health in six states. *American Journal of Preventive Medicine*, 11(6): 36–40.

Richards, TB, Rogers, JJ, Christenson, GM, Miller, CA and Taylor, MS (1995b) Evaluating local public health performance at a community level on a state-wide basis. *Journal of Public Health Manage Practice*, 1(4): 70–83.

Rillon, EB (2000) *Total Quality Management and Continuous Quality Improvement*. Manila: UPM.

Rimer, BK, Glanz, DK and Rasband, G (2001) Searching for evidence about health education and health behaviour interventions. *Health Education & Behavior* 28: 231–248.

Rosen, L, Rosenberg, E and McKee, M (2010) A framework for developing an evidence-based, comprehensive tobacco control program. *Health Research Policy and Systems*, 8: 17.

Rossi, P and Freeman, H (1985) *Evaluation: A Systematic Approach*. Beverley Hills, CA: Sage.

Rychetnik, L, Frommmer, M, Hawe, P and Shiell, A (2002) Criteria for evaluating evidence on public health. *Journal of Epidemiology and Community Health*, 56: 119–127.

Sackett, DL, Rosenberg, WMC, Gray, JAM and Richardson, WS (1996) Evidence base medicine: what it is and what it isn't. *British Medical Journal*, 312: 71–72.

Sackett, DL, Strauss, S and Richardson, WS (2000) *Evidence-Based Medicine: How to practise and teach EBM*, 2nd edition. Edinburgh: Churchill Livingstone.

Salcedo Aguilar, F, Martínez-Vizcaíno, V, Sánchez López, M, Solera Martínez M, Franquelo Gutiérrez, R, Serrano Martínez, S *et al.* (2010) Impact of an after-school physical activity program on obesity in children. *Journal of Pediatrics*, 157(1): 36–42.

Salmon, WC (1998) Scientific explanation: causation and unification, in Salmon, WC (ed.) *Causality and Explanation*. New York and Oxford: Oxford University Press.

Schünemann, HJ, Oxman, H, Brozek, J, Glasziou, P, Bossuyt, P, Chang, S *et al.* (2008) GRADE: assessing the quality of evidence for diagnostic recommendations. *Evidence Based Medicine*, 13: 162–163.

Scriven, M (1998) Minimalist theory of evaluation: the least theory that practice requires. *American Journal of Evaluation*, 19: 57–70.

Scutchfield, FD, Hiltabiddle, SE, Rawding, N and Violante, T (1997) Compliance with the recommendations of the Institute of Medicine report, The Future of Public Health: a survey of local health departments. *Journal of Public Health Policy*, 18: 155–166.

Shaneyfelt, T, Baum, K, Bell, D, Feldstein, D and Houston, T (2006) Instruments for evaluating education in evidence-based practice. *Journal of American Medical Association*, 296: 1116–1127.

Shavelson, RJ and Towne, L (eds) (2002) *Scientific Research in Education*. Washington, DC: National Research Council, National Academy Press.

Sheldon, B. and Chilvers, R. (2000). *Evidence-based Social Care: A Study of Prospects and Problems*. Dorset: Russell Housing Publication.

Silverman, D (2010) *Doing Qualitative Research*. London: Sage Publications.

Sim, J and Wright, C (2000) *Research in Health Care. Concepts, Designs and Methods*. Chelternham: Stanley Thorne.

Smith, SC, Lamping, DL, Banerjee, S, Harwood, R, Foley, B. *et al.* (2005) Measurement of health-related quality of life for people with dementia: development of a new instrument (DEMQOL) and an evaluation of current methodology. *Health Technology Assessment*, 9(10): 1–93.

Spooner, F and Browder, DM (2003) Scientifically based research in education and students with low incidence disabilities. *Research and Practice for Persons with Severe Disabilities*, 28: 117–125.

Staley, K (2009). *Exploring Impact: Public Involvement in NHS, Public Health and Social Care Research*. Eastleigh: INVOLVE.

Taylor, R, Reeves, B and Ewings, P (2000) A systematic review of the effectiveness of critical appraisal skills training for clinicians. *Medical Education*, 34: 120–125.

Taylor-Powell, E and Henert, E (2008) Developing a logic model. Teaching and training guide. University of Wisconsin-Extension. Cooperative Extension. Program Development and Evaluation. www.uwex.edu/ces/pdande/evaluation/evallogicmodel.html (accessed April 2011).

Thomas, J and Harden, A (2008) Methods for the synthesis of qualitative research in systematic reviews. *BMC Medical Research Methodology*, 8: 45.

Trinder, L and Reynolds, S (2000) *Evidence-Based Medicine: A Critical Appraisal*. London: Blackwell Publishing.

US Department of Health and Human Services (DHHS) (2008) *Consensus Statement on Quality in the Public Health System Public Health Quality Forum – 2008*. US Department of Health and Human Services Office of Public Health and Science Office of the Assistant Secretary for Health.

Ware, JF (2010) SF-36 Health Survey updated. www.sf-36.0rg/tools/sf36.shtml (accessed 26 December 2010).

Watterson, A and Watterson, J (2003) Public health research tools, in Watterson, A (ed.) *Public Health in Practice*. Houndsmill: Palgrave Macmillan, pp.24–51.

Wood, E (2003) What are extended matching sets questions? *Bioscience Education*, 1: 1–18.

World Health Organization (2001) *Macroeconomics and Health: Investing in Health for Economic Development*. Report of the Commission on Macroeconomics and Health. Geneva: World Health Organization.

World Health Organization (2002) *The World Health Report 2002. Reducing Risks, Promoting Healthy Life*. Geneva: World Health Organization.

World Health Organization (2006) *Immunization Costing and Financing. A Tool and Users Guide for Comprehensive Multi-Year Planning (cMYP)*. Geneva: World Health Organization.

World Health Organization (2009) *WHO Guide to Identifying the Economic Consequences of Disease and Injury*. Department of Health Systems Financing. Geneva: World Health Organization.

World Health Organization (2003) *Health Systems Performance Assessment: Debates, Methods and Empiricism*. Geneva: World Health Organization.

Index